# FIT 4 THE FIELD

## A FITNESS GUIDE FOR THOSE WHO HUNT, FISH AND TRAP

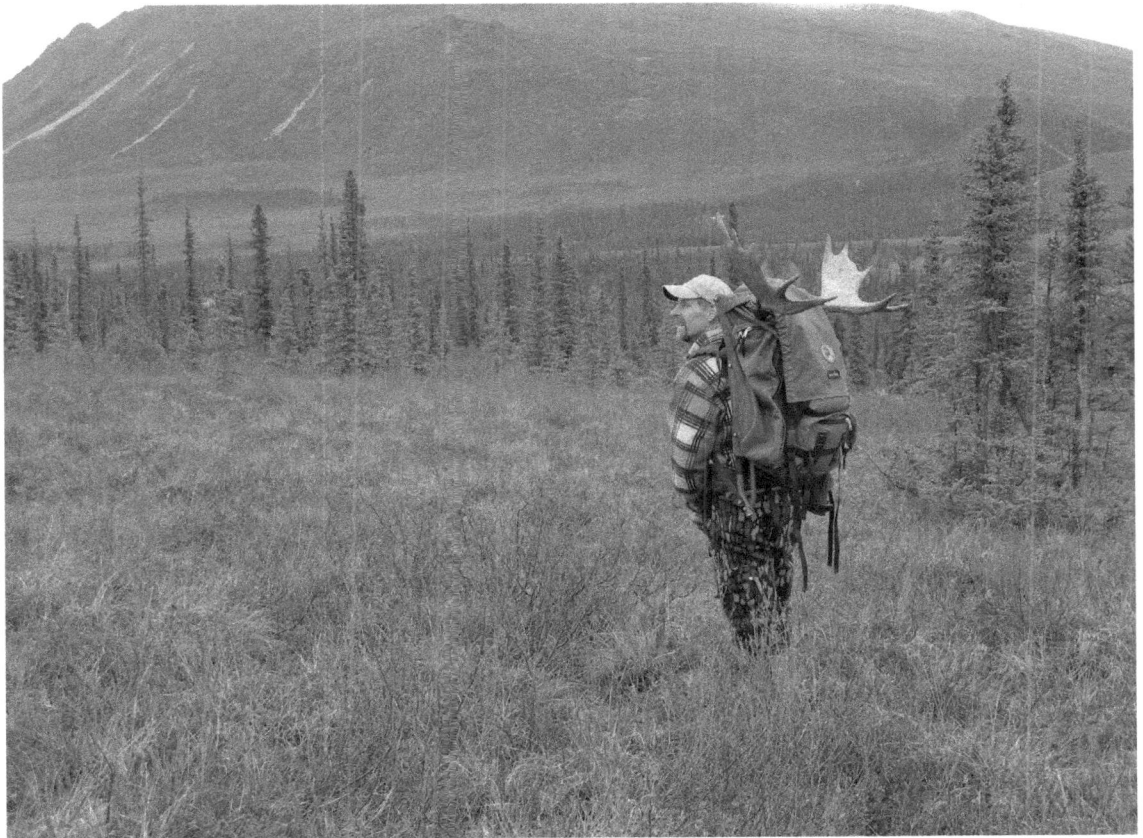

## GRANT HILDERBRAND, PH.D.

Published by
Spartan Fitness Press


The Publication Arm of
Spartan Fitness Alaska, LLC
5800 Kalgin Drive
Anchorage, AK 99516

Fit 4 The Field: A Fitness Guide For Those Who Hunt, Fish, and Trap

Design by Adrienne Wilkerson © January 2011
Beacon Publishing & Design, LLC. www.beacon-design.com


ISBN 13: 978-0-9841784-2-1
ISBN 10: 0-9841784-2-2

# TABLE OF CONTENTS

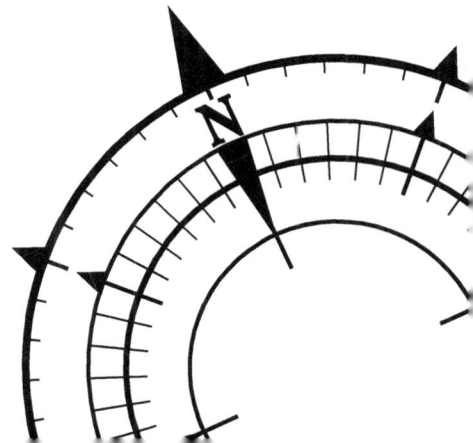

# ACKNOWLEDGEMENTS

This book is the result of the efforts and encouragement of so many of my friends and colleagues. This collaboration is, without question, what made this project so enjoyable and rewarding. In particular, I want to thank Tom Paragi, Sally Guynn, Gina Main, Steve Belinda, and Cathie Harms for helping to shape the concept and reviewing the manuscript. The book is far better for their time and efforts. Mike Tietjen, Doug Larsen, Layne Adams, Nick Demma, Dwight Guynn, Sally Guynn, Tom Vania, Dave Rupp, Jon Heggen, Terri Stewart, and Gino Del Frate graciously shared photos that did far more than my words to illustrate the usefulness of fitness to sportsmen. I also want to thank Troy Jarvis, Marten Martensen, Kris Burnett, Sean Gange, Mike Anderson, and Brent Eaton. They helped with the exercise photos and, even more important, are my workout partners that continue to push me further than I would push myself. Three local gyms in Anchorage warrant special recognition: Southside Strength and Fitness, Alaska Functional Fitness, and Pete's City Gym. Finally, I want to thank my family for their love and encouragement. Thank you.

# DEDICATION

*For my grandfather, Curtis Hilderbrand - thanks for letting me nip at your heels in the sticks and hollows*

*"You must invest in your fitness
so that your body responds
appropriately when called upon"*

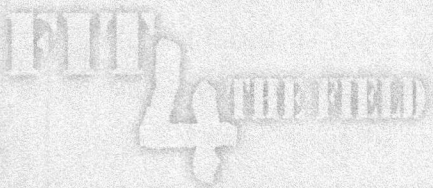

# CHAPTER 1:

## THE OUTDOOR SPORTS PERSON AS ATHLETE

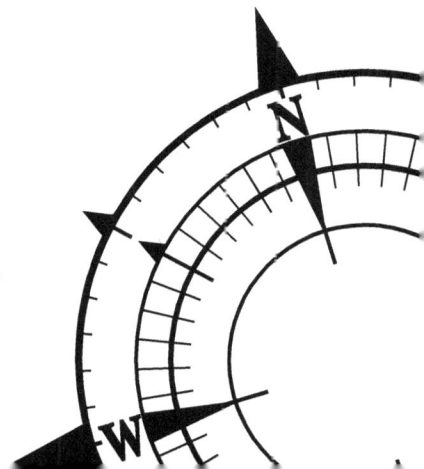

When you think of the word athlete, what comes to mind? For many, it will be those individuals that participate in popular spectator sports such as football, baseball, hockey or basketball. Some may think of Olympians of the past or present that excel at fundamental activities such as running, jumping, or sparring. Today, an appropriate definition includes golfers, skateboarders, snowboarders, bull riders, and dancers.

Common to all those who excel in the varied activities above is their effective application of knowledge, skill, and physical ability to complete a task or challenge. Using this as a working definition, those who hunt, fish, trap, or otherwise recreate in the outdoors can clearly be defined as athletes.

Athletes can improve their overall performance by increasing their capacities in any of these three areas. Many of the most successful quarterbacks excel on the field because of the time they invested in the film room during the week studying the common schemes and formations used by their opponents. They look for tendencies that can provide an advantage and are able to apply these insights when standing at the line of scrimmage. Similarly, a golfer prepares by studying and practicing on a particular course, making mental note of the lie of the greens, the length of the grass, and the

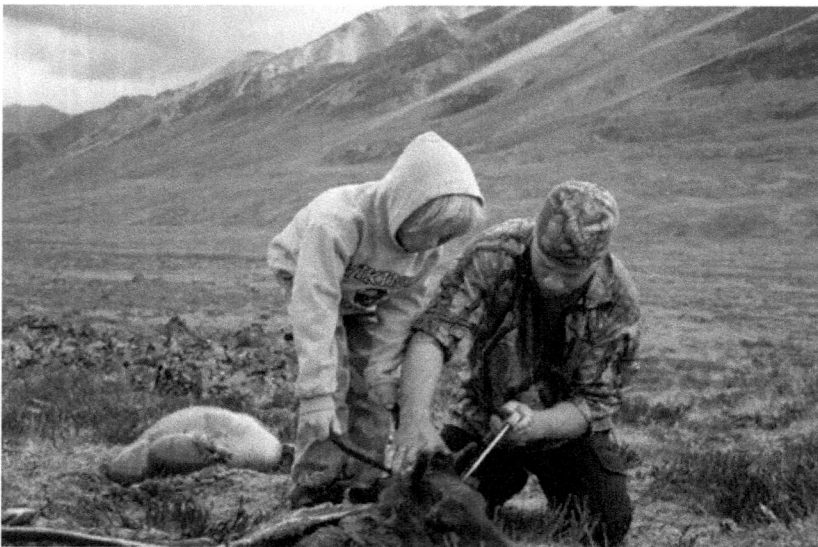

pattern of the winds. This preparation leads to increased knowledge which enhances their performance in a competitive event.

Skills are critical components of many athletic endeavors. Baseball pitchers and soccer players continually practice and improve their ability to modify the path of the ball. In both events, the ability to create unpredictable speeds and flight paths provide a competitive advantage. This ability is the product of developed and practiced skills.

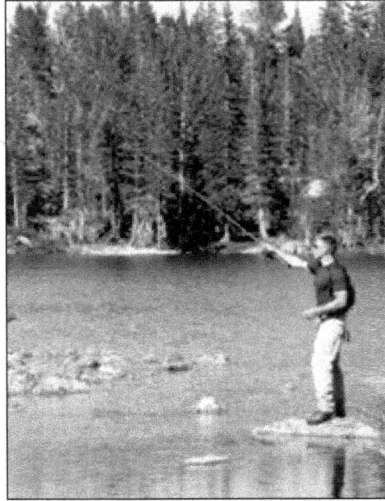

The linkage between one's physical prowess and one's athletic performance is fundamental. The strongest, fastest, most agile athlete starts from a position of advantage. Those less gifted or less physically trained start at a disadvantage and strive to use knowledge and skill to close the gap. The point is that anyone who seeks to maximize their performance in any athletic event should strive to address all three key elements of athletic performance: their knowledge, their skill, and their physical capacities.

This brings us back to the outdoor sports person—fishers and hunters. To be successful in our pursuit of fish or wildlife, we must know the habits of our prey. Dedicated hunters, anglers, and trappers acquire a voluminous knowledge of the life history, behavior, habitat preferences, reproductive patterns, and seasonal activities of the fish or game they pursue. Outdoorsmen and women study the water and land where they fish and hunt, learning it like the back of their hand. They invest significant time increasing in their knowledge with the intent of increasing their efficiency, effectiveness, and, ultimately, their likelihood of success.

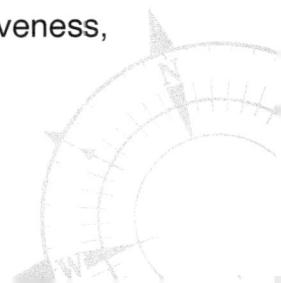

Whether fishing with a fly rod or a spear gun or hunting with black powder, bow, or rifle, you have to develop specific skills to be effective at harvesting prey. Not only are you likely to be unsuccessful without adequate practice, it would be irresponsible to pursue game unless you had developed the skills necessary to quickly and humanely kill that which you pursue.

The physical demands faced by sportsmen are significant and diverse. Hiking long distances across uneven terrain carrying a pack, climbing into a tree stand, striding from one rock to another crossing a stream, ducking under or hopping over a downed limb, paddling a canoe across a current, fighting a 600 lb marlin on a boat deck which rolls with the waves, or managing the weight of big game during butchering all require strength, endurance, and agility.

A sportsmen's ability to perform these tasks safely is paramount. Unlike athletes competing in the controlled environment of stadiums or manicured courses, medical assistance for sportsmen faced with minor or major injuries may be hours or even days away. What may be insignificant in an arena can be life-threatening in the field. Physical training will reduce your chance of injury should you

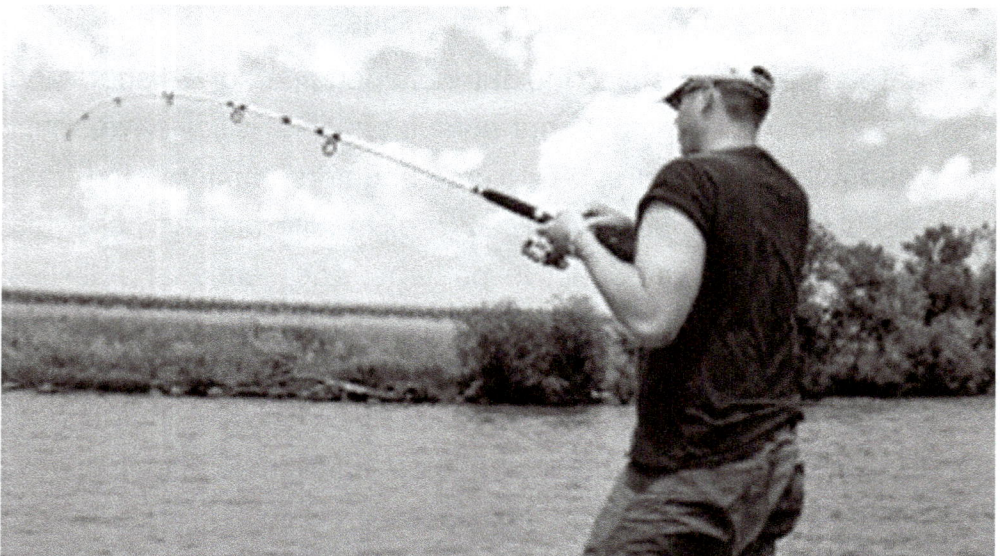

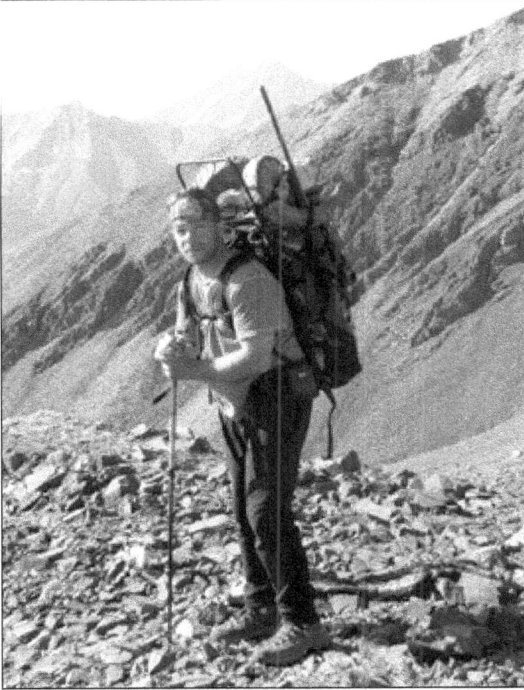

trip, slip, or fall. What's more, a broad approach to fitness that includes balance, agility, and coordination work as well as aerobic, anaerobic, and strength training exercise will make you less likely to stumble in the first place.

Sportsmen and women invest significant resources in the tools they use to harvest fish and game. A good gun or top-end fly rod can cost thousands of dollars. These items are also diligently cared for and maintained so that their performance when called upon is reliable and effective. Just as with a rifle or bow, the sportsman's body is a critical tool. You must invest in your fitness so that your body responds appropriately when called upon.

Hunting, fishing, trapping, and other outdoor recreational pursuits are lifelong activities. Your ability to participate and enjoy these pursuits late into life depends on your fitness. These activities are also indelibly linked to family. The knowledge necessary to successfully harvest deer, turkey, bass, or beaver is most often passed from grandparent to parent and parent to child. Similarly, many of us were taught to shoot or cast by our mom or dad or grandma or grandpa. Dedication to physical fitness benefits you. But is also sets an example for your children and grandchildren. Remaining healthy and physically active as you get older is part of your legacy. It is a responsible investment in future generations.

*"A fitness without walls"*

# CHAPTER 2:

## AN ORGANIC APPROACH TO FITNESS

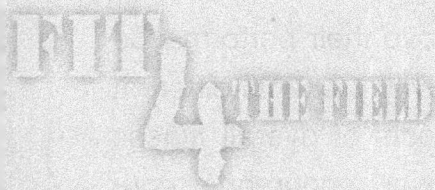

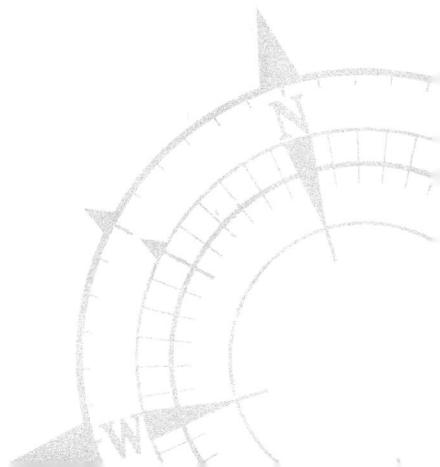

Relative to your health, the reasons to exercise are innumerable. Everything from your heart to your bones to your hormone levels to your joints to your digestion to your mental acuity benefits from regular physical activity. You live longer and you live better. This is reason enough to dedicate yourself to maintaining and enhancing your fitness.

One reason individuals train is to improve their performance in a particular event or sport. While each activity presents different physical demands, several fundamental aspects of overall fitness are constant across all athletic pursuits: power, endurance, core strength, balance and agility, flexibility and range of motion, and kinesthetic awareness – an innate sense of your body in space relative to your environment.

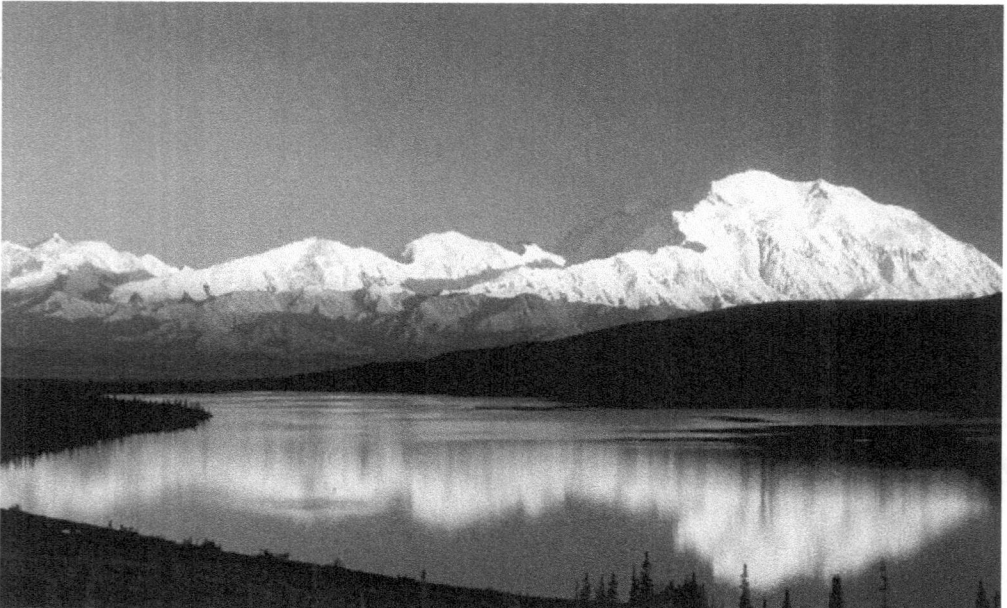

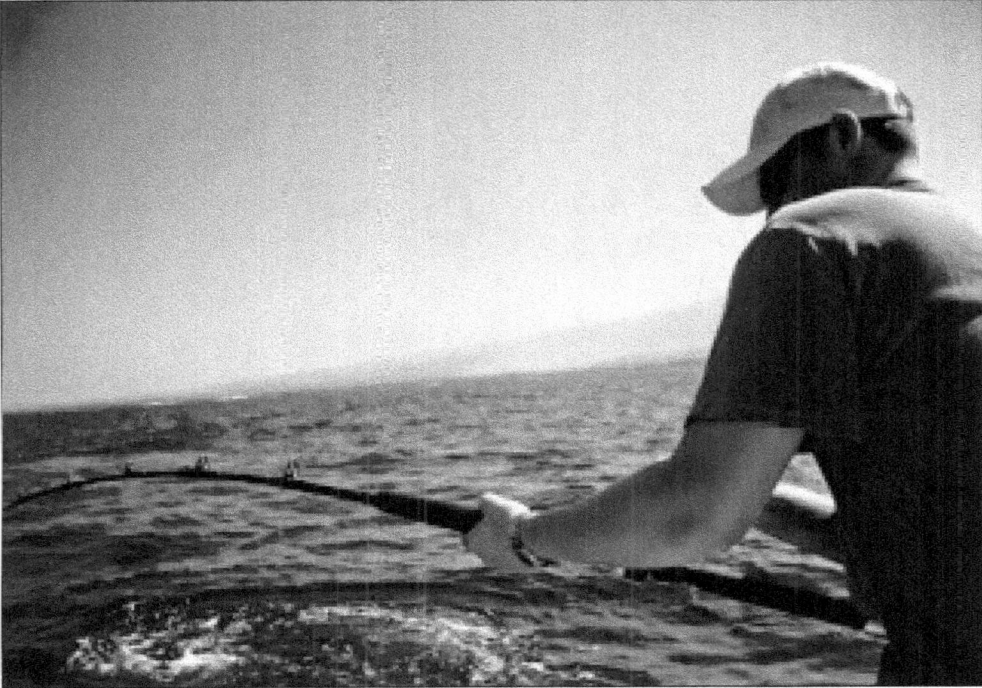

As an athlete, you need to address all of these aspects of your fitness. Further, you need to address them in a way that serves you well in the activities in which you participate. Tremendous work has been done developing and refining the appropriate exercise regimes for common sports such as football, track and field, baseball, soccer, etc. Aspects of these programs serve the sportsman well. However, the sportsman faces two key additional challenges: diversity and variability.

In the game of baseball, some games are played in the day and some are played at night. Occasionally, the game is played indoors instead of outdoors or on field turf instead of natural grass. But there is always 90 feet between the bases. The environment is always largely controlled. The same is true of most organized sports.

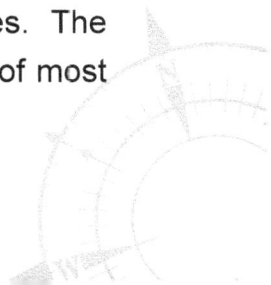

## Mosaic Construct of Fitness

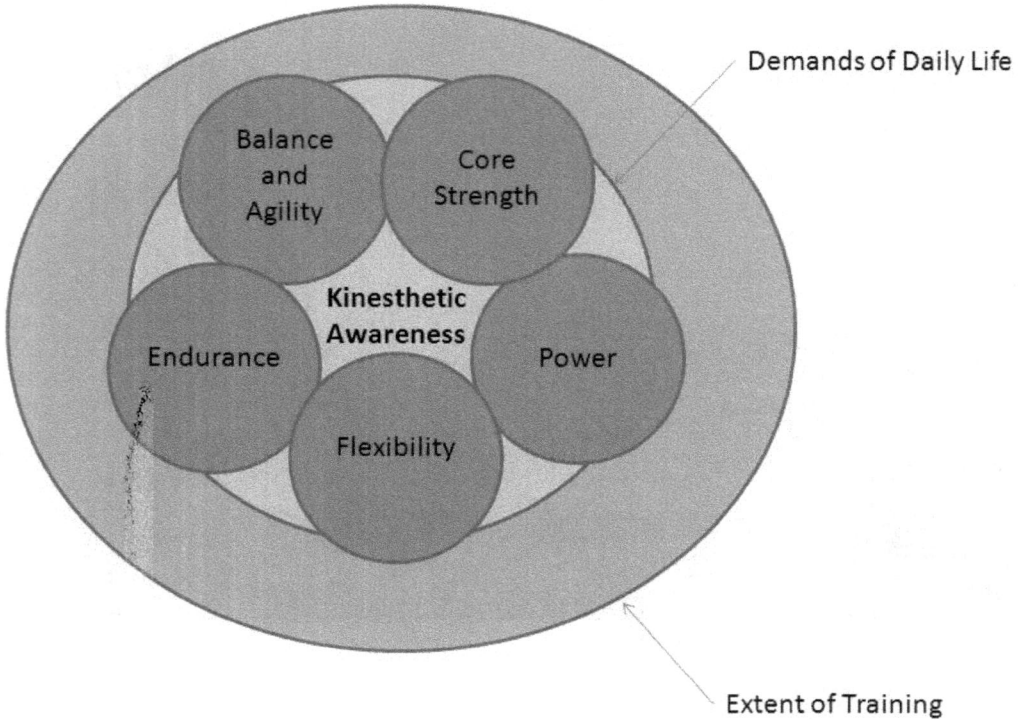

Balance and Agility

Core Strength

Demands of Daily Life

Kinesthetic Awareness

Endurance

Power

Flexibility

Extent of Training

I've spent more than 20 years working as a wildlife biologist, mostly in Alaska. I love the outdoors. I've never had much use for a world with walls. When I began working in the fitness field, the majority of my clients were non-traditional athletes. They hike and climb and canoe and kayak and ski and fish and hunt. Depending on the time of year, their focus shifts. The range of physical challenges and environmental conditions they face are as varied as their interests. Thus, the fitness I pursue for myself and for my clients is a fitness that translates well once you leave the temperature controlled gym and step off the pavement - a fitness without walls. This broad concept of fitness recognizes the import of cardiovascular and muscular endurance (aerobic capacity), power (anaerobic capacity), range of motion, as well as agility and balance. This definition acknowledges that these fitness categories form an overall mosaic and attention must be paid to each component.

Training in the gym benefits functional capacity by allowing us to fully and efficiently develop all components of our overall fitness; however, we are striving for a fitness that matters not only in the gym, but in daily life when you lift a bag of dog food, pick up your child or grandchild, or climb a ladder to clean the gutters. Further, we are looking for capacities and abilities that translate to the mountain, the trail, or the water  Functional fitness has to address your ability to participate and succeed in daily life and in the activities you enjoy. It has to improve your quality of life.

We will train all the fitness elements listed above.  However, we will blur the lines between the categories.  We will focus on large body functional movements that develop your ability to generate and control significant power.  These movements simultaneously enhance your endurance due to the heavy oxygen demands of your working muscles.  By learning proper technique, building strength, and increasing range of motion, we will reduce your likelihood of injury.  Full body movements have two additional advantages.  They condition the core muscles of the abdomen, lower back, and hips and develop agility and balance.

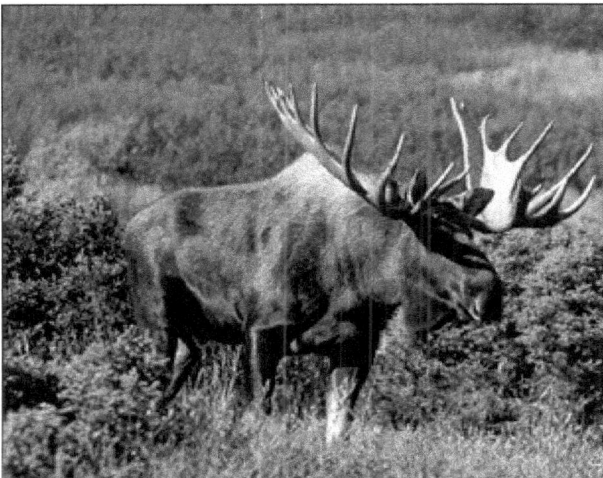

We will also dedicate specific attention to coordination and kinesthetic awareness. These aspects of fitness are critical when you get off the groomed trail and have to navigate obstacles and variable terrain. We all have friends or family members that have sustained serious injuries to their bones or joints while recreating in the outdoors. Accidents happen. But when you head in the field, you have a certain level of responsibility to your hunting or fishing partners. If you are prone to injury, you can contribute to bad situations that can compromise their safety as well as your own. Similarly, if a member of your party becomes injured, you should possess the physical prowess and basic training to capably care for him or her until help can arrive or you can get them to safety.

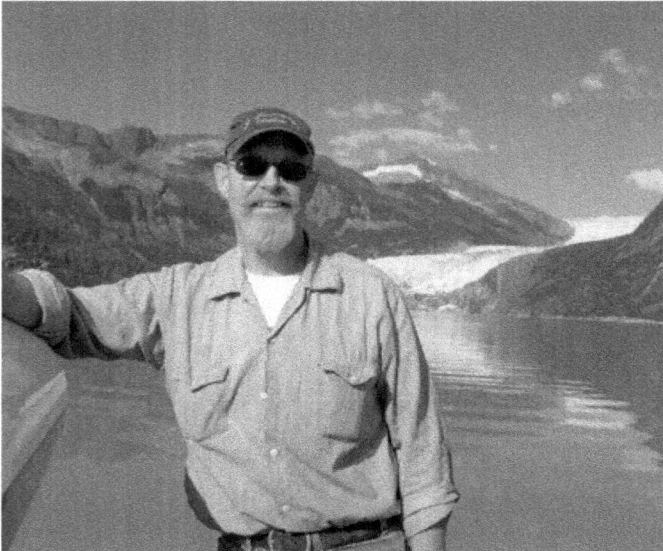

The exercises in the following chapters are challenging, but they all have an underlying practicality. Together, they will develop a mosaic of fitness that will prepare you for anything. Your fitness is dynamic, changing through time. It can be shaped and honed. Left unattended, your fitness will deteriorate; however, with proper effort it can be improved and refined regardless of age. My intent is to prepare you for the diversity and unpredictability that lays in wait in the world of the sportsman.

In chapters three to seven, I describe fundamental exercises that will foster improvement in power (Chapter 3); endurance (Chapter 4); core conditioning (Chapter 5); coordination, balance, and agility (Chapter 6); and flexibility and range of motion (Chapter 7). While each of these exercises has been explicitly categorized into a single chapter, realize that most benefit multiple fitness components simultaneously. This is precisely why they are useful for developing an integrated, functional fitness. Throughout, pay strict attention to form, because proper execution is critical to your ability to do the exercises efficiently and safely.

This list of exercises is meant to be representative and is by no means exhaustive. As a trainer, I constantly watch, ask about, and try new exercises. I am always looking for new tools that I can use in my own workouts and with my clients. I don't want to imply any ownership of the exercises covered in this book; I am only endorsing them.

*"Power is the product of coordinated strength and speed"*

# CHAPTER 3:

## POWER

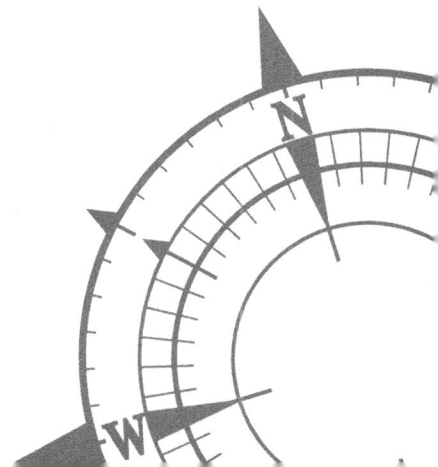

Practically speaking, strength is the ability to exert force, speed is the rate of motion, and power is the application of force over time and distance. In essence, power is the product of coordinated strength and speed. Functionally, power is largely what we use in everyday life. Power is how you set a hook, heave a bag of feed into the back of your truck, and lift a canoe from the ground onto your shoulders for portage. We want to train for power, not just for strength.

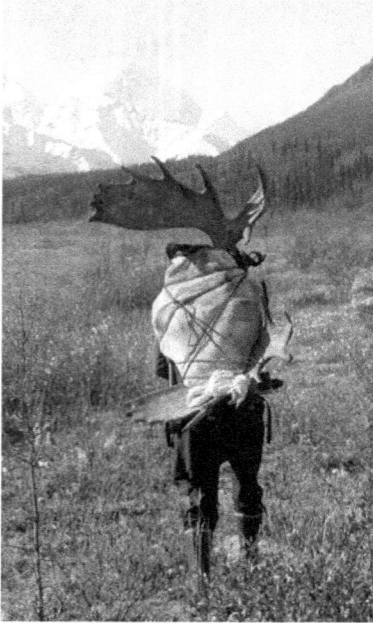

We want to focus on developing power that translates outside the gym. To do so, we will replicate functional movements. This will train the body to move, generate inertia, and handle momentum the way it was designed. Your body doesn't function as a collection of independent muscles and joints clumsily handing work from one body segment to the next like a bucket brigade fighting a fire. Instead, the body very fluidly and very efficiently transfers power generated in large muscles to smaller and smaller muscles. It is a highly orchestrated series of fulcrums and lever arms that can execute an endless variety of tasks in multiple planes. Further, training and using the body as designed is less likely to result in strains or other injuries; whereas imbalances can result from isolation training.

Rarely do practical movements span a single joint. Further, they commonly occur in multiple planes (i.e., involve not only forward and backward movements, but rotation as well). As an example, envision the way your body moves when splitting logs with an axe or maul. Strength is required to lift the axe overhead. But, the speed and strength generated by the hips and core are what result in the tremendous power transferred to the head of the axe and delivered to the log. The ankle, knee, and hips of the lower body are all engaged and the body's core and upper body play important roles in stabilization, balance, and momentum transfer. Finally, there is significant body rotation, thus the movement occurs in multiple planes.

Almost any athletic movement requires motion across multiple joints and occurs in multiple planes. Similarly, many muscle groups have partners that balance and support complex actions. These muscle groups are called force couples (e.g., the bicep and triceps, the abdominals and lower back, the hamstring and quadriceps) and their complementary training both enhances performance and reduces the risk of injury by preventing one muscle from overpowering another. For this reason we will largely avoid the simple isolation movements and machines common to traditional body-building regimens (e.g., bicep curls, leg extension machines, hamstring curls). To develop functional power we largely want to select exercises that replicate, or at least enhance practical movements that span multiple joints. Further, we want to include some work that requires the generation and control of power in multiple planes typical for movements and activities by outdoorsmen and women.

# STRENGTH TRAINING BASICS

Many people find their first visit to a weight training facility overwhelming. The multitude of machines, clanging weights, and grunting, sweaty lifters can make it hard to know where to start and, for some, be intimidating.

This is unfortunate as weight training has significant health benefits ranging from maintaining or increasing muscle mass and

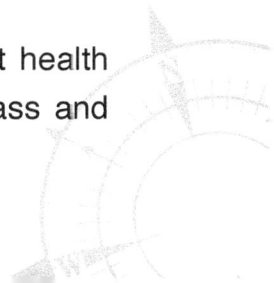

bone density to increasing basal metabolic rate to improving aerobic and anaerobic conditioning.   Further, resistance training enhances core strength, agility, balance, and body awareness.  For these rea-sons, strength training should be part of any fitness program for any-one at any age.

Despite the number of machines, racks, platforms, and weights, there are just a few basic categories of movements you need to know to begin effective training:

1. Isolation movements: these movements focus on one particular muscle group.  Their benefit largely lies with body building or post-injury rehabilitation.  I rarely include isolation movements in client training programs.  You can always identify movements by counting the number of joints that move during the movement.  Isolations have only one moving joint and a common example is a bicep curl as the only movement occurs at the elbow.

2. Complex movements: these movements include multiple muscle groups that complement each other and are used functionally in everyday life and recreational activities.  When you observe complex movements, you will be able to identify at least two moving joints.  There are 3 sub-categories of complex movements:

   a. Pressing movement with the legs:   there are a variety of movements (squats, dead lifts, lunges) and machines (leg press, hack squat) that train this movement.  In all cases, you are using your legs to either press something away from you or press yourself away from something.  Movement typically occurs at some combination of the ankle, knee, and hip.

   b. Pulling movement with the upper body:  Any time you pull something towards your body or pull your body towards some-thing, you are executing a pulling movement.  Pulling movements can be done throughout the 180 degrees spanning the front of the body ranging from pulling directly over head (e.g., a pull up) to pulling an object from the waist to shoulder height (e.g., an upright row). When pulling, movement occurs at some combination of the elbow, wrist, shoulder, and shoulder blade.

c. Pushing movement with the upper body: These movements are simply the reverse of the pulling movements discussed above. They involve the same joints and occur in the same 180 degree span in front of the body. You can always match a pushing movement with a pulling movement (e.g., a lat row and chest press, a pull up and a shoulder press). [poling a canoe upriver]

3. Compound movements: these movements combine two or more complex movements. Generally, they involve generating power below the waist and then transferring this power through the core where it can assist an upper body movement. Due to the large size of the muscles of the legs, hips, and buttocks, they can significantly assist the smaller upper body muscles and the coordinated utilization of these different muscle groups is both natural and functional. Examples of compound movements are cleans, push presses, and thrusters.

Gyms are commonly equipped with dumbbells, barbells, plates, cables, medicine balls, kettle bells, and a variety of machines. If you observe others using this equipment or experiment with them yourself, you will find that they are almost always appropriately used for one of the three types of movements described above. Further, there are numerous ways to train the same muscle group. As an example, the large muscles of the chest can be trained by doing pushups, by using a chest press machine, by doing bench presses with a barbell, or by doing chest flies with dumbbells. Across these tools, the movement and muscle groups trained are virtually the same.

Generally, one progresses from machines to barbells to dumbbells, though many advanced athletes will continue to utilize all of these tools. Machines largely dictate your form as they only allow movement in the appropriate direction and plane. In addition, they focus only on the muscle group targeted and do not rely on core or non-target muscles for balance or stabilization. After developing basic strength and a kinesthetic awareness of the proper movement patterns, individuals can progress to more advanced tools and exercises that challenge balance and coordination and develop core strength.

The benefits of strength training are numerous, thus strive to include them in your fitness program. After a little practice, any intimidation or trepidation you may have will fade. Further, always feel free to ask gym staff, trainers, or other members for guidance or clarification if you have any questions. We all learned at some point and most people will be happy to help you out.

Below I describe the fundamental power training movements.

# SQUATS

The squat is the single most fundamental functional movement of the human body. It is how you get up and how you get down. I recommend the squat as the foundation of any fitness programs for any purpose at any age. You can squat heavy (e.g., 300+ lbs on a barbell on your back) or light (e.g., a medicine ball or just your body weight) and see endless benefits. It allows movement over multiple joints and is particularly effective at developing the functional ability to generate and transfer power from the hips. Envision climbing upslope with a pack when putting a stalk on a band of sheep and packing out meat after a successful hunt. The power you are able to generate and apply is greatly enhanced by squats. This is true on both the ascent, where you must lift the weight of your body and gear against gravity, and the descent, where you must control your weight and external load as you lower it to prevent injury. Because of the number of large muscles engaged and resulting increased oxygen demands, squats can provide cardiovascular benefits as well.

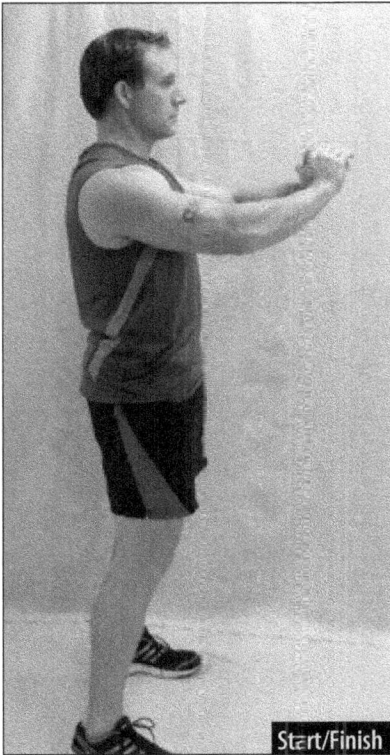

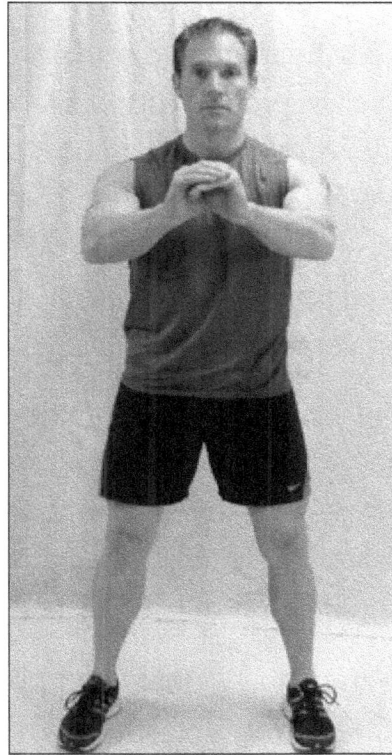

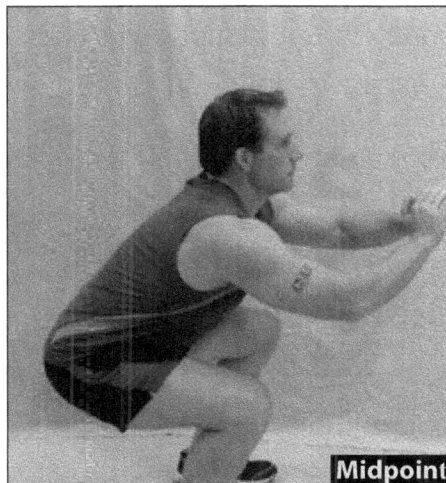

Start/Finish

Midpoint

## COACHING POINTS

1. Develop a stable base. Your feet should be just wider than shoulder width apart with your feet turned out 5° to 10°.

2. The weight should be centered directly over your lower leg (i.e., you should neither be on your toes nor on your heels).

3. Your head should remain level throughout the entire motion as this will protect your back by ensuring correct posture. If training with a mirror, focus your gaze on your reflection roughly at the level of your forehead. If no mirror is available, pick a point at eye level on the facing wall. Whether using your reflection or another guiding mark on the wall, maintain visual contact throughout the movement.

4. Your initial movement should be down and back with your hips, not forward with your knees. To help envision the correct movement, imagine that someone has a rope tied around your waist and is pulling you from behind simultaneously backwards and down.

5. With heavy weight, your depth should be as low as you can go, while being able to comfortably return to a standing position. With light or no weight, go as deep as you are able and strive to increase your range of motion over time (see Chapter 7 for a more detailed discussion of squat depth).

6. Your upward movement is initiated by a powerful press against the floor. Envision trying to push the floor away from you. This initial press is smoothly, yet powerfully transferred to the hips. Here, envision bumping a door closed using your hips.

7. Throughout the movement, your core will remain contracted and your normal, upright back posture should be maintained.

8. Breathe in during the downward phase and out during the upward phase.

# DEAD LIFTS

The dead lift is an often underappreciated and, unfortunately, underused exercise. People think dead lifts aren't for everyone as they tend to envision power lifters straining to lift bar-bending loads. In functional terms, a dead lift is the appropriate way to pick up any object from the ground, everything from a child to an outboard motor to a cooler full of freshly caught fish. Similar to the squat, it has significant benefits for the development of hip and leg generated power, has significant cardiovascular benefit due to the large muscle groups engaged, and can be performed with heavy or light weights.

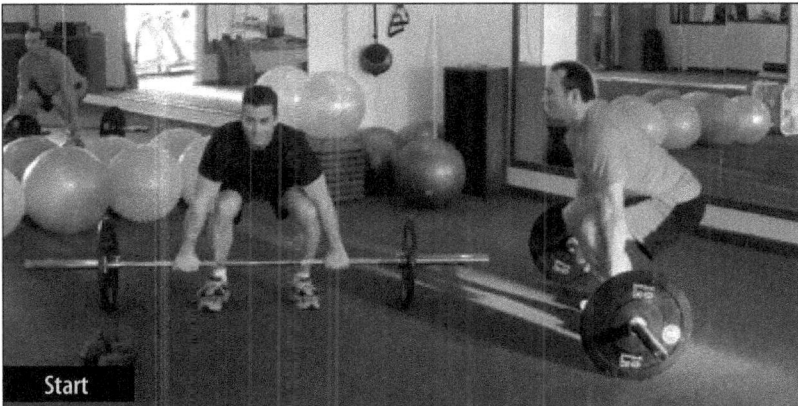

Start

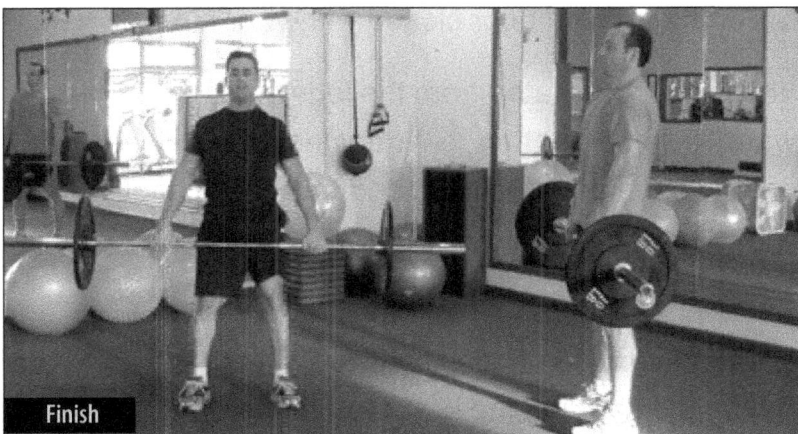

Finish

## COACHING POINTS

1. Develop a stable base. Your feet should be slightly narrower than a squat, roughly shoulder-width apart with your feet turned out 5° to 10°.

2. The distribution of weight across your foot should be centered directly over your lower leg (i.e., you should neither be on your toes nor on your heels—you should be able to wiggle your toes throughout the duration of the movement).

3. Your head should remain upright with your gaze directed slightly below eye-level throughout the entire motion as this will protect your posture. Imagine a penny on the ground roughly fifteen feet in front of you and keep your eyes on this penny as you execute the lift. You don't want your head straining upward or bending downward.

4. Your arms should be straight and vertical, in line with the weight, and perpendicular to the floor.

5. Your initial movement should be initiated with the legs, largely the butt (gluteus) and thigh muscles (quadriceps and hamstrings). Envision powerfully pushing the floor away from you.

6. As you move the weight upward, the hips become engaged. Envision bumping a door closed with your hips.

7. As the power generated from the legs and hips drives the weight upward, the momentum will transfer to the upper back (latisimus) and shoulders (deltoids and trapezius) and you will roll the weight slightly back through your shoulders to a position of control.

8. The weight can then be lowered to the floor in the reverse order with the legs carrying the majority of the burden on the descent.

9.  Be sure to maintain good posture on the descent as well as the lift.

10. The weight should be touching or nearly touching your body throughout the entire movement.

11. Breathe in during the downward phase and out during the upward phase.

# LUNGES

Lunges are an exaggerated stepping motion that challenges the upper thigh muscles of each leg independently. Lunges enhance lower body power, range of motion, and muscular endurance in activities such as hiking or running on variable terrain. Further, the lunge movement requires significant balance, relying on the muscles of the lower leg and the lateral and medial muscles of the hips and thighs. This is extremely useful in activities like back country skiing for recreation or to check a trap line as skiing requires not only leg power but also balance to maintain the long, effective glide on alternating skis. Lunges can be performed using one's body weight, medicine balls, dumbbells, or barbells. In addition they can be performed in a forward stepping motion, stepping backwards, or at a slight angle to involve the inner and outer thigh muscles.

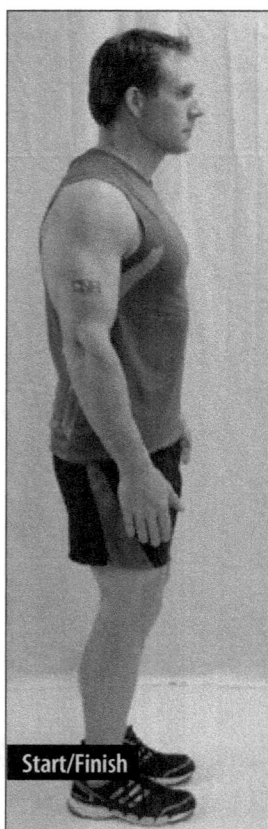

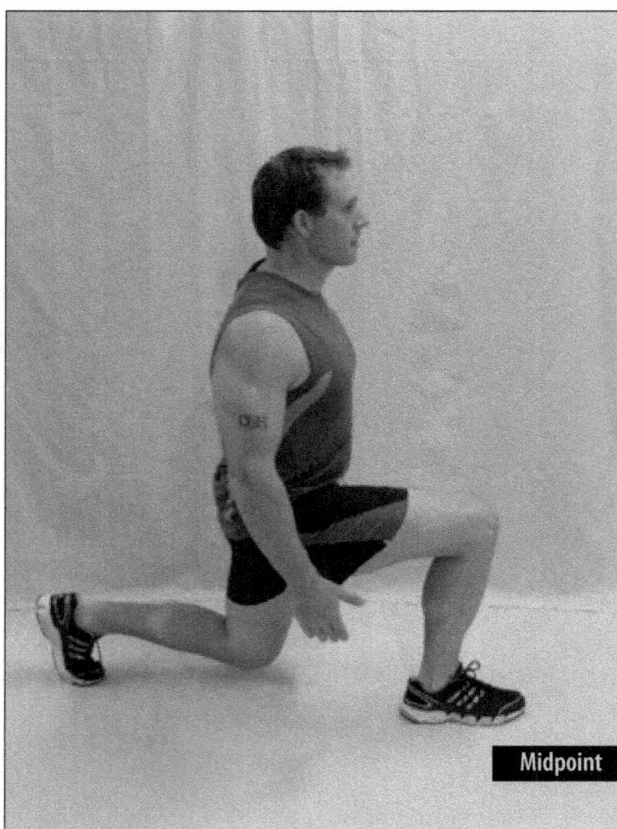

Start/Finish

Midpoint

# COACHING POINTS

1. Your stance should be similar to your normal standing position.

2. As you step forward, you want your stride to be slightly longer than normal, resulting in a 90° angle between the upper and lower leg of your forward leg, a 90° angle between the upper part of your forward leg and your torso, a 90° angle between your two upper legs, and a 90° angle between the upper and lower leg of your trailing leg.

3. Do not exaggerate the movement. Thus, do not hyperextend the trailing hip or allow the knee of the forward leg to move forward of the foot.

4. This movement involves both a forward step and then a controlled down and up motion.

5. The legs should be the primary muscles used to control your descent and drive the ascent.

# CALF RAISES

Calf raises complement the power developed through squats, dead lifts, and lunges by utilizing the full range of motion at the ankle joint and strengthening the muscles of the lower leg. Calf raises will also enhance balance, especially at full extension of the foot. Calf raises can be performed on any step or platform and working through the full range of motion will help maintain elasticity in the Achilles tendon, thus reducing the likelihood of tears. Strengthening of the small muscles of the lower leg will help prevent sprains as well.

## COACHING POINTS

1. Stand such that your toes are securely placed on the surface but your mid-foot and heel movement are unimpeded.

2. Raise and lower your body in a slow and controlled manner through the full range of motion at the ankle.

3. Foot placement (toes pointed slightly inward, slightly outward, or straight ahead), external weights, and one leg raises can be used to provide variation and increased intensity.

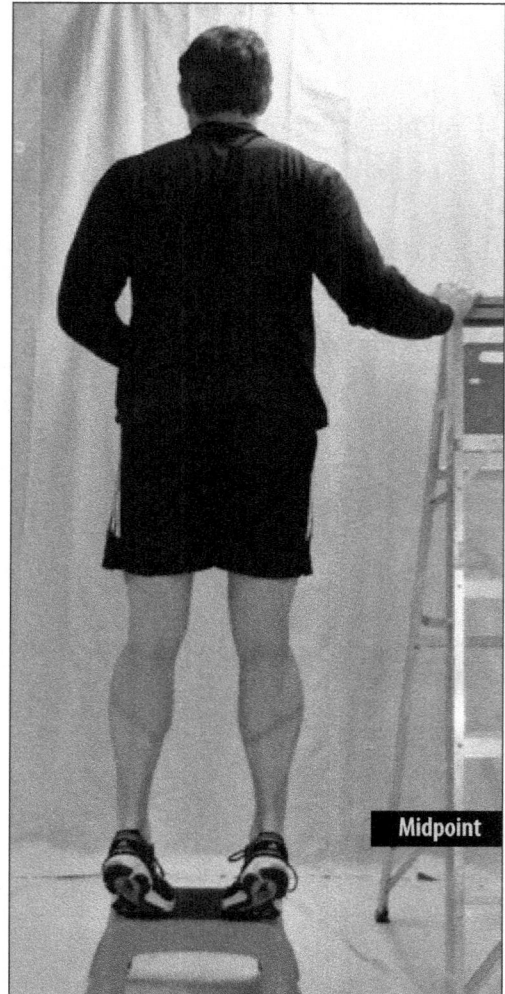

Midpoint

# PULL-UPS/LAT PULL-DOWNS

Pull-ups are an outstanding exercise that engages all of the upper body muscles functionally used to pull (i.e., lift) your body mass against gravity. Any type of climbing or swimming benefits greatly from enhanced upper body strength developed through a pulling motion. Use of an overhead pulley to hang your harvest utilizes a similar movement. Specifically, the large muscles of the back (latisimus) are the major movers with assistance from the shoulders (rear deltoids, trapezius) and the front of the upper arms (biceps). Because many individuals can not complete a large number of repetitions using their body weight, assisted pull-ups and/or lat pull-downs can be used to tra n the same muscles through the same range of motion, but with reduced resistance.

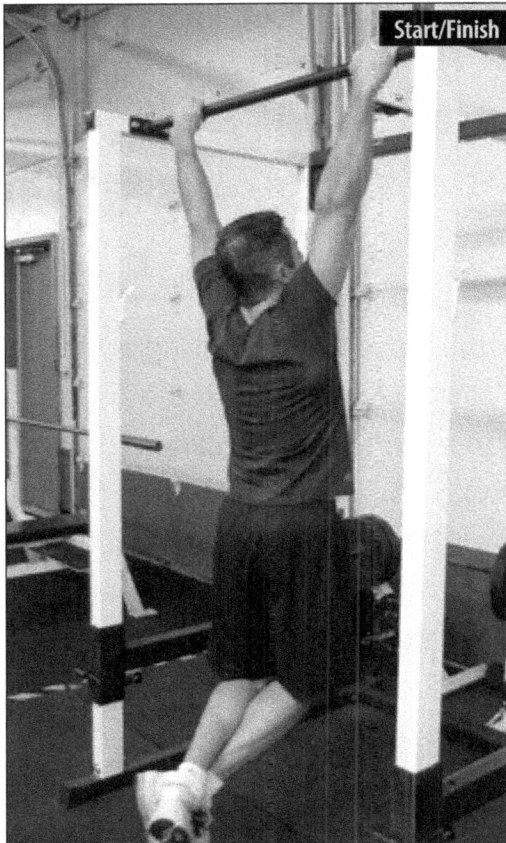

Start/Finish

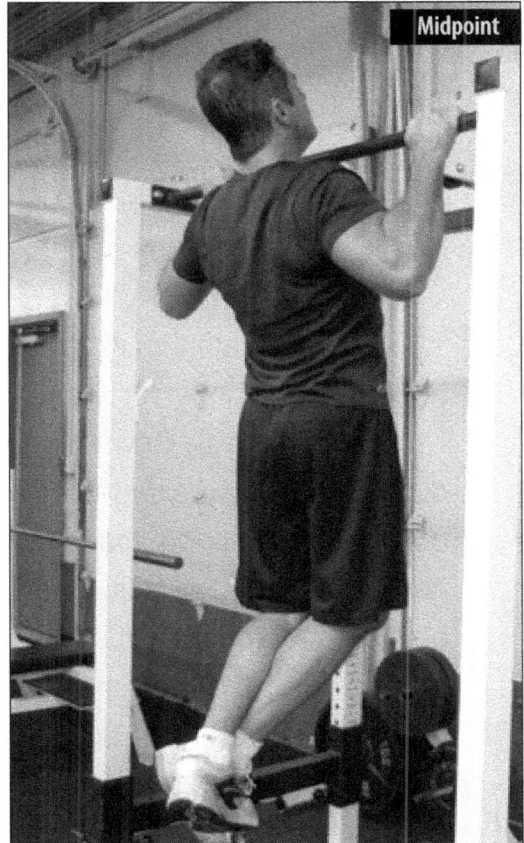

Midpoint

## COACHING POINTS (PULL-UPS/LAT PULL DOWNS)

1.  Start from the downward position and allow yourself to relax your shoulder blades and hang, fully stretching your back and shoulders.

2.  A variety of grips can and should be used over time.

3.  Initiate the movement with the large muscles of the back. This momentum should then be smoothly transferred to and built upon first by the shoulders, then by the arms.

4.  Continue the movement until your chin clears the bar.

5.  After a momentary pause, lower yourself in a controlled manner to the full, stretched downward position.

6.  Allow momentum to cease and repeat the movement.

# ROWS

Rows train you in the functional movement of pulling an object towards your body (or your body towards an object if the object is heavier than you). Rows can be done in a variety of planes (perpendicular to gravity or against gravity), with a variety of tools (dumbbells, barbells, cable machines, etc.). Depending on the angle to the ground and the direction of pull, different muscles can be emphasized but the primary movers are the large muscles of the back (latisimus), the muscles of the shoulder (deltoids and trapezius) and front of the upper arm (biceps). This exercise certainly benefits any activities (e.g., drawing back a bow, kayaking or canoeing) or movements (e.g., turning over a pull-start motor, sawing wood) that require this specific movement. In addition, strength developed in this plane will balance strength gained through pull-ups and through the pressing movements described below. Utilizing a variety of approaches is recommended.

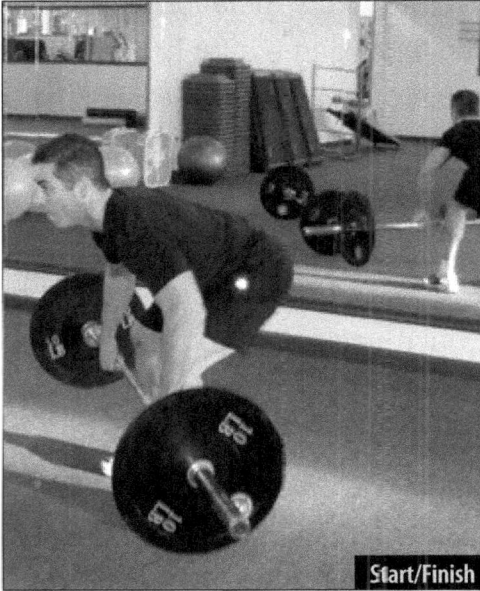

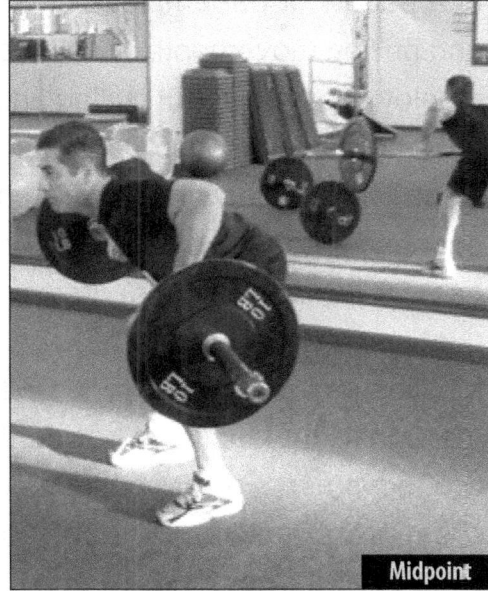

Start/Finish          Midpoint

## COACHING POINTS (ROWS)

1. When performing standing upright rows, your stance should be similar to that of a squat with your feet slightly wider than shoulder width and your knees slightly bent to protect your lower back.

2. Ensure a full stretch of your back when extended.

3. Initiate the movement with the large muscles of the back (latisimus); thus the first movement should be in your shoulder blades, not your shoulders or arms.

4. Finish the movement by fully contracting the back. Envision trying to hold a pencil between your shoulder blades.

# PUSHUPS/BENCH PRESS

The pushup and bench press functionally replicate the natural action of pushing an object away from you or pushing yourself away from an external object. In canoeing and kayaking, the use of a paddle or oar employs the coordinated combination of pushing and pulling movements. Maneuvering large game after harvest often employs both powerful pulling and pushing movements. Power in the pushing motion is also important to other activities such as the efficient use of poles when cross country skiing. The primary muscles engaged are those of the chest (pectorals), shoulders (deltoids), and back of the arm (triceps); however, due to the balance required by pushups and chest presses, additional muscles of the core and legs function as active stabilizers. Collectively, these muscles can generate significant functional power. The primary difference between the two movements is that pushups control one's body weight while the chest press requires control of an external object. Numerous variations exist for both movements including incline and decline bench press. Pushups can be modified by varying hand width, using grips to increase depth (i.e., range of motion), or resting on one's knees to reduce the resistance.

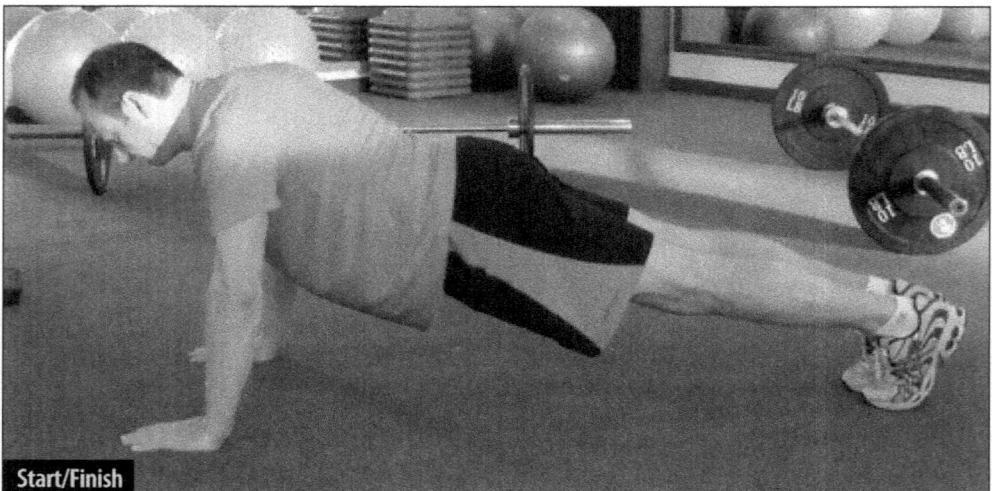

Start/Finish

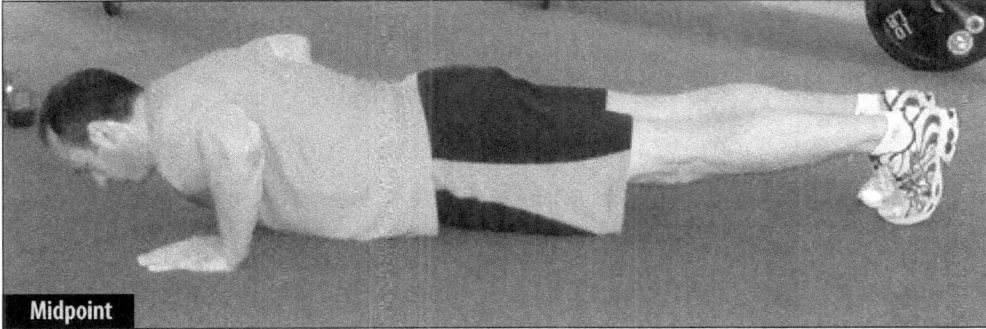

Midpoint

## COACHING POINTS (PUSHUPS/BENCH PRESS)

1. Focus on a stable base.

2. If doing pushups, your body should be a solid plank from the top of your head through your heels throughout the movement.

3. If doing presses lying on a bench, ensure your head, shoulders, and glutes are in contact with the bench throughout the movement. Similarly, keep your feet flat on the floor to balance your body.

4. During the negative movement (i.e., the barbell or the floor coming towards you), the angle of your elbow should break (be less than) 90°. When using a barbell, the bar should touch your chest roughly at a line drawn between your nipples. You should inhale during the negative phase.

5. The pressing movement (i.e., the barbell or floor is moving away from you) should be initiated by the muscles of the chest (the pectorals) rather than by your shoulders or arms.

6. When finishing the movement, straighten your arms to engage the back of the upper arm (triceps).

7. As a reminder, breathe out during the pressing movement.

# SHOULDER PRESS

The shoulder press functionally allows one to lift an object overhead. The primary muscles utilized are the shoulders (deltoids) early in the movement and the back of the upper arm (triceps) late in the movement. Shoulder strength is important in a wide variety of activities ranging from lifting to climbing to rowing to skiing. In addition to enhancing performance, developing shoulder strength and range of motion has significant value in injury prevention as this joint is susceptible to painful and slow-healing strains and sprains. Either barbells or dumbbells can be used to execute this functional movement and, ideally, it is performed in a standing position as this actively engages the core body muscles as stabilizers and more closely mimics practical movements.

## COACHING POINTS

1. Use the same stance as for squats with a slight bend in the knees to protect the lower back.

2. Throughout the movement, keep your wrist, elbow, and shoulder in line vertically to ensure efficient lifting effort.

3. When elevating the weight, fully press the weight upward such that your shoulder blades and shoulders are fully extended, as if reaching for the sky. Exhale when pressing the weight upward and inhale during the downward phase.

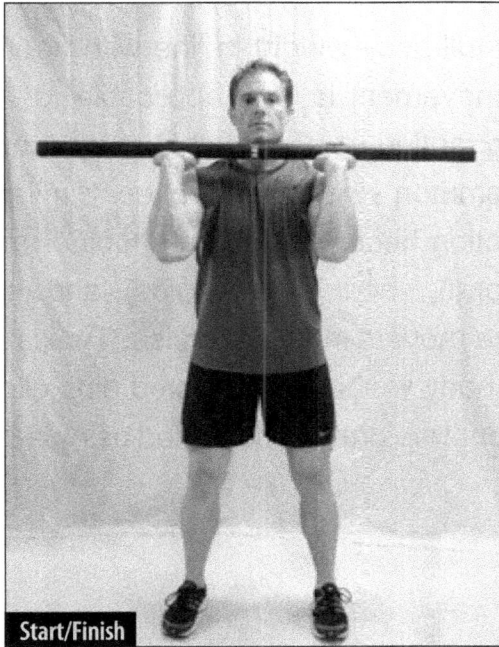

Start/Finish

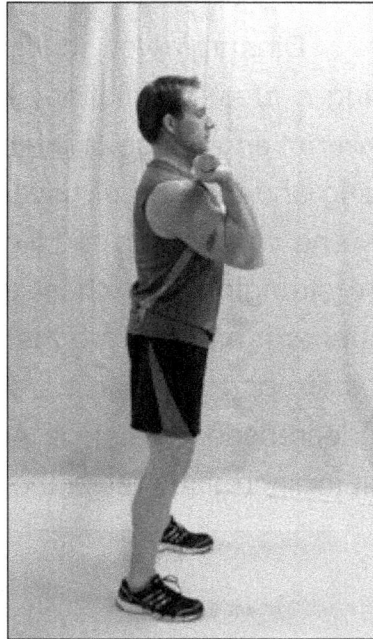

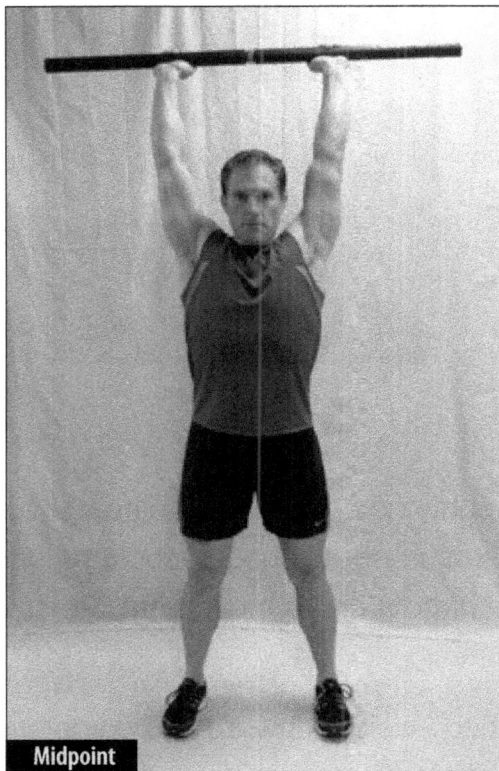

Midpoint

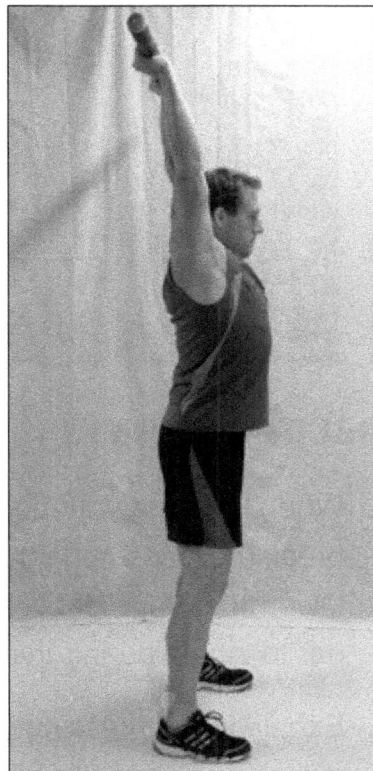

# DIPS

Dips train you to lift your full-body weight in line with gravity using a pressing motion. This movement is very applicable to the powerful end phase of the poling motion used by both cross country skiing and the end of several common swimming strokes. Similarly the end of a strong paddling motion heavily relies on shoulder and arm strength. Your chest (pectoral), shoulders (deltoids), and rear upper arm (triceps) are the active movers in this exercise. Typically, dips are performed using one's body weight but assisted dips allow for decreased resistance. Additional weight can be added using a hip belt for increased resistance.

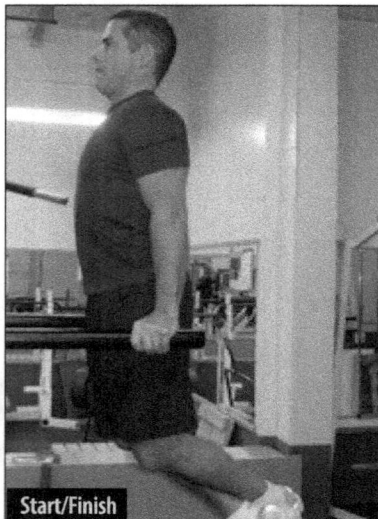

Start/Finish

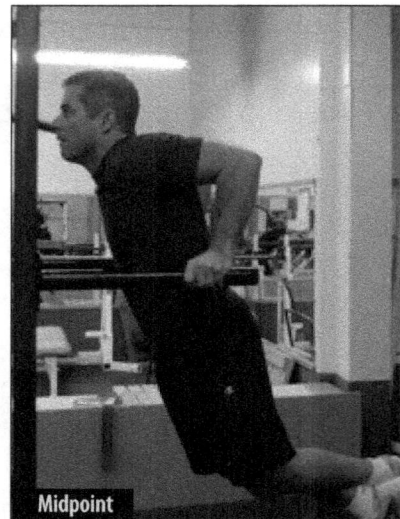

Midpoint

## COACHING POINTS

1. When lowering your body weight, the angle of your elbow should break (be less than) 90°. The result is your shoulder being slightly lower than your elbow at the bottom of the movement. Remember to inhale during this phase.

2. Exhale when pressing your body weight upward and completely extend your arms to fully engage your triceps.

# FULL BODY MOVEMENTS

The following three exercises combine multiple individual functional movements. The advantage of practicing these movements is their real world practicality (i.e., lifting an object from the floor to chest height and then overhead). For example, imagine lifting your canoe from the ground to an overhead position for shoulder portage or having to right a capsized boat, snow machine, or ATV. Further, because they require the use of large muscle groups of both the upper and lower body, significant oxygen is required, resulting in aerobic and anaerobic benefit. The core muscles of the body are actively and functionally engaged as they serve not only to stabilize, but also transfer power from the lower body to the upper body. Finally, practicing compound movements is beneficial to overall coordination and body awareness. In essence, connecting the movements connects the body.

# POWER CLEANS

The functional use of the power clean is lifting a relatively heavy object from the ground to the chest position, such that your arms are underneath the object, allowing you to place the object or lift it overhead. It is, in essence, a dead lift coupled with a squat. My fifteen-year-old dog, Mickey, continues to accompany me on outings, but his aging hips require that I lift him into and out of the back of my truck. In essence, this is a 70 lb power clean. This is a very effective movement that is both practical and offers significant training benefit.

## COACHING POINTS

1. Start in a dead lift position after reviewing the dead lift coaching points provided earlier in this chapter.

2. As the hips engage, driving the weight upward, initiate a shoulder shrug. However, rather than the shrug lifting the weight higher, use the shrug to pull yourself under the weight.

3. As you pull yourself under the weight, arrive in a squat position such that the weight is securely held by your hands with your arms underneath and in control of the weight. The weight should be located roughly at the height of your collarbone.

4. Execute a squat to finish the movement.

5. When the movement is complete, return to the beginning dead lift position.

6. During the entire movement, keep the weight close to your body. The path the object follows should be as vertical as possible.

7. Control your breathing throughout the movement due to the high oxygen demands.

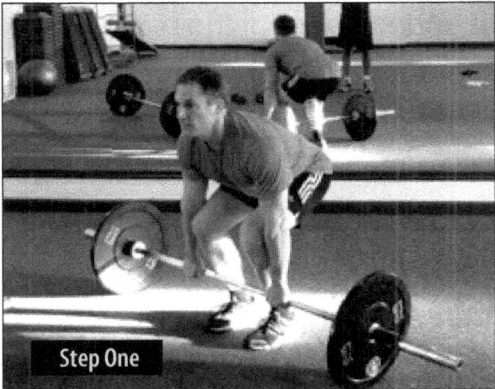

Step One

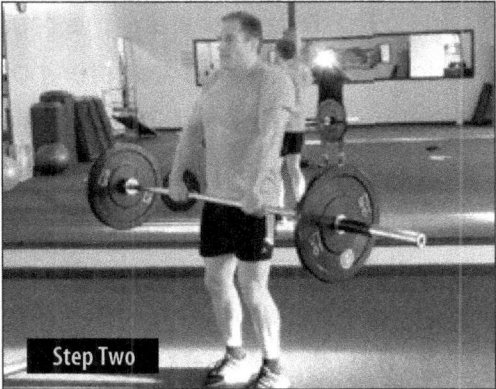

Step Two

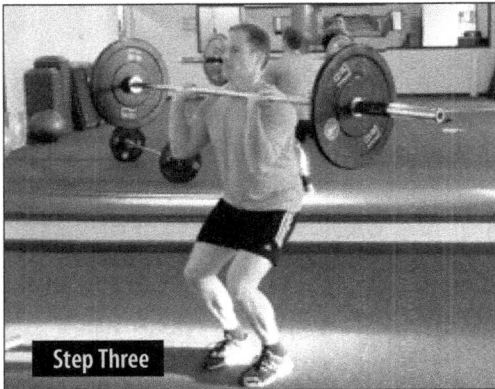

Step Three

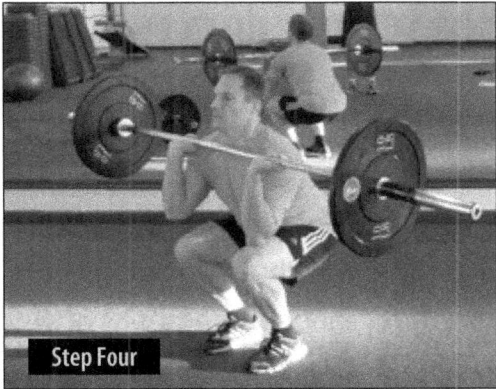

Step Four

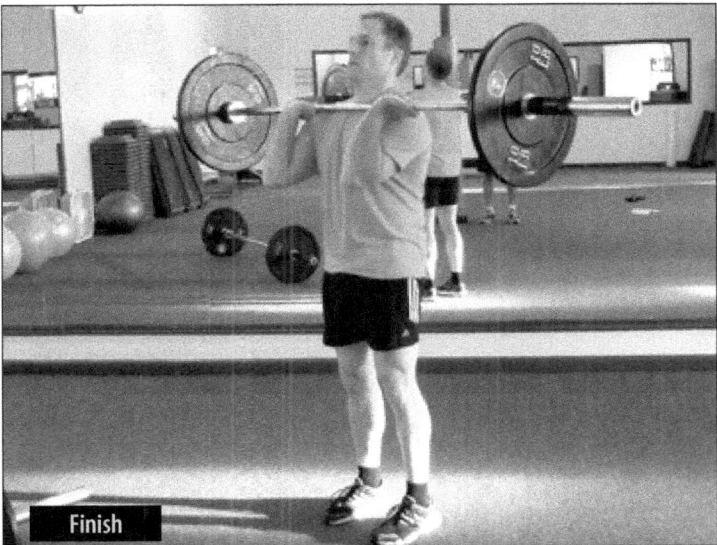

Finish

# PUSH PRESSES

Push presses are the result of engagement of the hip flexors, which generate and transfer power to a shoulder press. Most individuals can safely lift 2–3 times more weight overhead using a push press movement rather than a simple shoulder press. Functionally, this movement is the appropriate way to lift heavy objects from chest height to above the shoulder. Saddling a horse or mounting gear on your roof rack benefits from good form and functional power in the push press.

## COACHING POINTS:

1. This movement is identical to the shoulder press with one major exception.

2. The movement is initiated with a quick, explosive dip and drive of the hips that adds significant power to the movement and greatly increases the amount of weight that can be lifted overhead.

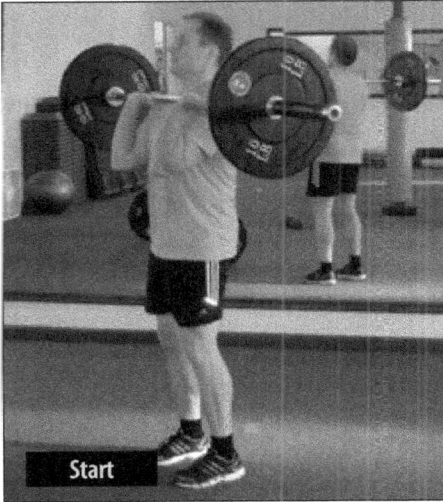

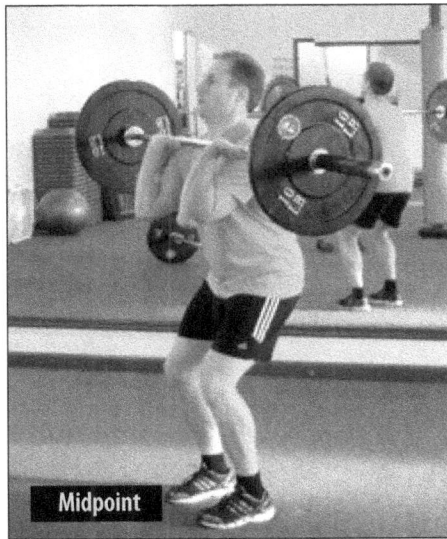

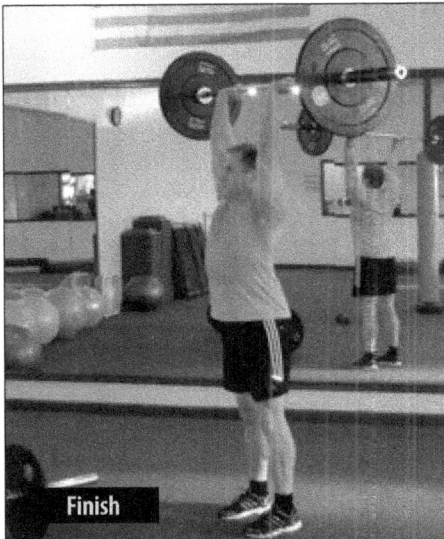

# THRUSTERS

A thruster is the combination of a squat with a shoulder press. The power initiated with the squat is carried through and added to by the shoulder press. It should be performed as one fluid movement rather than two distinct movements performed in sequence. A power clean combined with a thruster would be the appropriate way to move a heavy object from the ground to an overhead position (e.g., swapping a bin of winter gear for summer gear from the floor of your garage to an overhead shelf).

## COACHING POINTS

1.  Start in a downward squat position with the weight located at collarbone height. Your arms should be below the bar with your hands securely holding the weight.

2.  Just as with a squat, the movement is initiated powerfully with the legs followed by the hips.

3.  As the hips engage, the shoulder press is initiated resulting in a fully extended shoulder press.

4.  When performed correctly, the weight is elevated upward so powerfully by the legs and the hips that it almost floats upward and is largely weightless against the shoulders and arms until much of the shoulder press movement is complete.

5.  Similarly, if done properly, your feet will almost leave the ground.

6.  The path of the weight should be nearly vertical.

7.  Once in the upward position, reverse the movement, returning to the starting position with your legs receiving the weight.

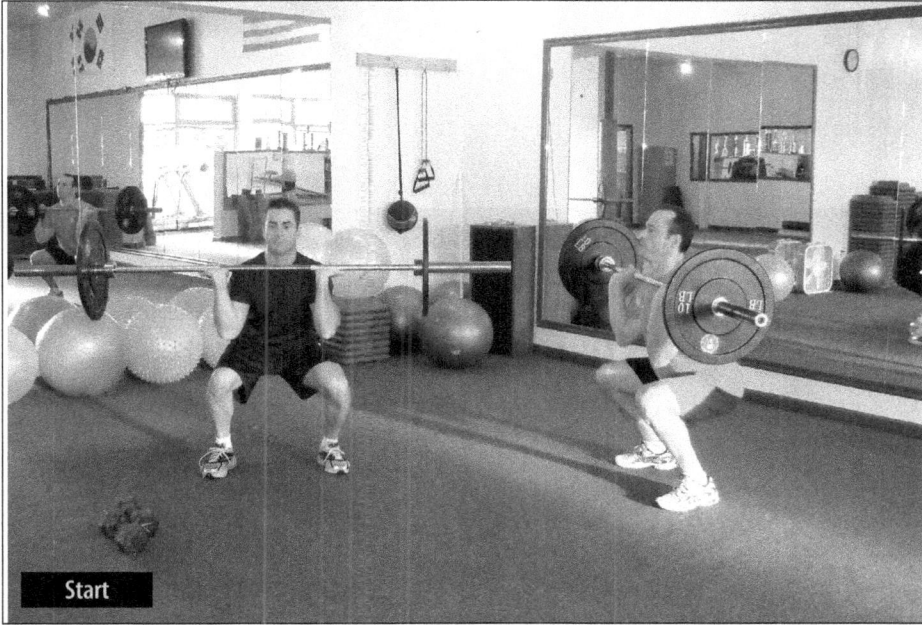

Start

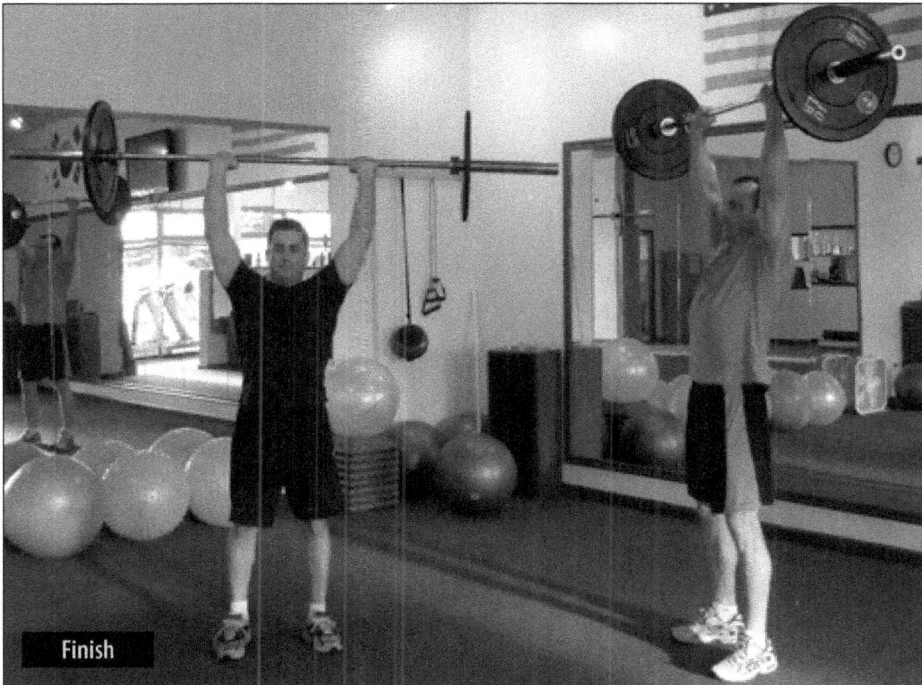

Finish

*"Efficiency can be improved
through training"*

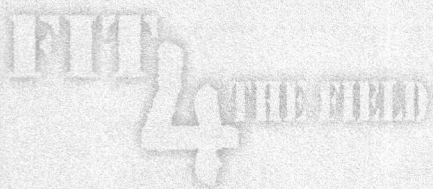

# CHAPTER 4:

## ENDURANCE

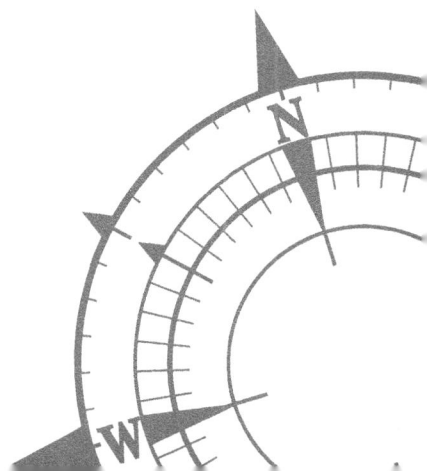

The term "cardio" usually refers to exercises designed to improve cardiac (i.e., heart) function. In essence, your body requires constant delivery of oxygen and nutrients to your working muscles as well as removal of metabolic byproducts. These transfers occur through the blood, which is delivered by the pumping action of the heart. These demands are increased during exercise and training benefits cardiac efficiency by increasing stroke volume (the amount of blood pumped per beat). Due to this increased efficiency, trained individuals have lower heart rates both at rest and during activity than untrained individuals. Despite the reduced heart rate, the increased stroke volume results in increased cardiac output (the amount of blood delivered per unit of time). At the cellular level, your ability to produce energy, carry and absorb oxygen, and eliminate waste improves. Ultimately, your efficiency is increased at multiple levels. Collectively, these efficiency gains result in improved performance.

Another way to look at endurance is in the broader context of the three metabolic pathways that supply energy for muscle contraction, since this is the ultimate function we are looking to improve through training. The aerobic energy system requires oxygen and utilizes glucose, fatty acids, and amino acids. The glycogen–lactic acid system does not require oxygen (i.e., is anaerobic)

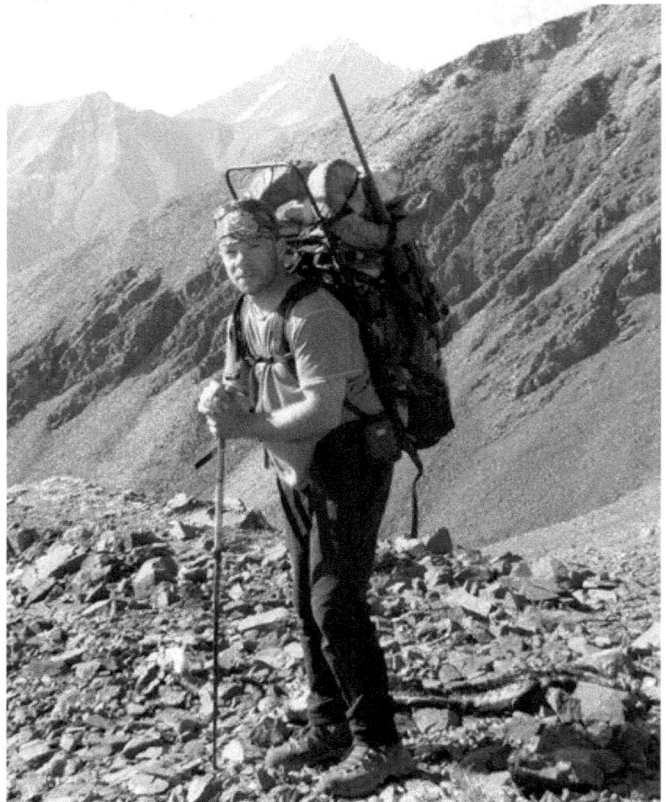

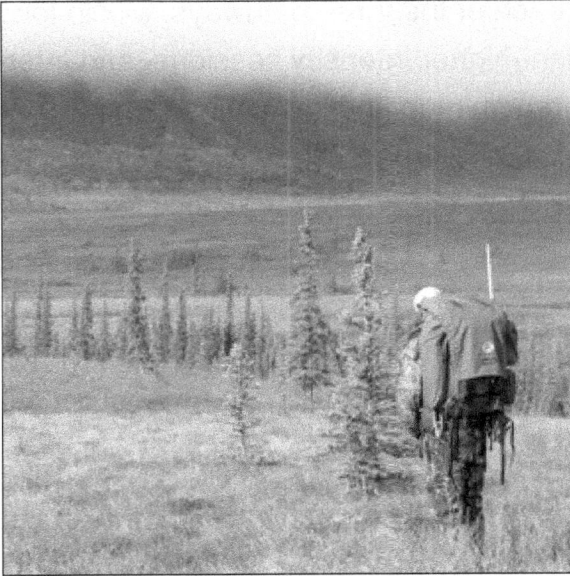

and utilizes glycogen stored in the muscles. Finally, the phosphagen energy system uses adenosine triphospate (ATP) and phosphocreatine and is also anaerobic.

From a functional standpoint, long duration, low intensity activities rely almost exclusively on the aerobic energy system. Very short duration (e.g., 10–15 seconds), high intensity (e.g., maximum squats) bouts of activity engage the phosphagen system. The glycogen–lactic acid system is utilized for activities that are intermediate in duration (30–40 seconds) and intensity. The glycogen–lactic acid system and the phosphagen system can provide energy very quickly, but the stores utilized are also limited and quickly depleted. The aerobic energy system requires some time to engage but the energy stores are more plentiful. Thus, lower intensity activities can be maintained longer. Additionally, only 20% of the energy released aerobically goes to support muscle contraction while the remaining 80% is released as heat.

The point critical to us is that the efficiency of all three pathways and, therefore, one's performance when tasking each pathway, can be improved through training. Further, whether hiking five miles on variable terrain to and from camp or engaging in an hour long battle while sport-fishing on open water, you rely on your endurance. Thus, we can and should include a wide variety of activities in our training. Further, we should vary the intensity and duration at which these activities are performed as an explicit part of our fitness program so that we address each of the three pathways. Mix in long slow sessions, shorter duration–higher intensity sessions, and interval sessions (single bouts with both high and low intensity; e.g., walk a block, jog a block, run a block, and repeat). This allows simultaneous training of both aerobic and anaerobic energy pathways.

There are endless possibilities relative to cardiovascular and muscular endurance training. Traditional exercises or approaches such as running/jogging, biking, swimming, rowing, etc., all have the potential to significantly improve cardio-respiratory function. We should especially include exercises that utilize multiple pathways simultaneously (e.g., skiing, hiking, or biking on variable terrain or canoeing or kayaking with, against, and cross current).

While all of these movements are, without question, functional, my recommendation is that one train in a variety of activities and mix in outdoor sessions as well. This will prevent the mental boredom that can come from over-structured or routine sessions. Developing competency in activities like climbing, skiing, and snowshoeing will broaden the tools available to you and allow you to maintain your fitness across the seasons, regardless of the climate you live in. Workout diversity reduces the likelihood of injuries resulting from

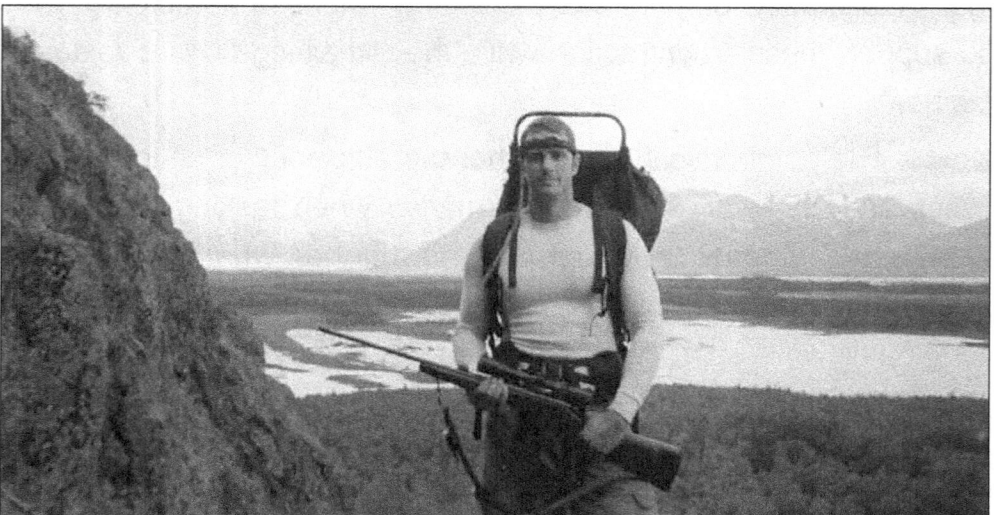

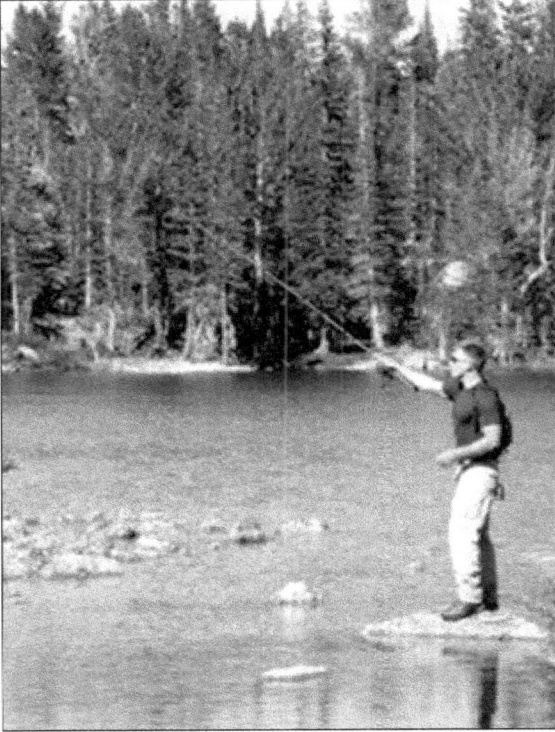

repetitive movements and fosters the flexibility bene-fits that come from engag-ing in a wide variety of activities through their full range of motion.

One common limita-tion most of us face is time. A functional and effective way to improve cardio-respiratory function is by performing the power exer-cises in the previous chap-ter and the agility and bal-ance exercises in Chapter 6 at high intensity. Intensity can be increased by reducing the rest time between sets, increasing the rate at which the exercise is performed (without compromising form), or increasing the resistance.

Whole body movements (e.g., power cleans, thrusters, push presses) are particularly effective in this regard due to the high oxygen demands of simultaneously engaging multiple large muscle groups. This approach to these exercises is, in essence, our holy grail as we are simultaneously training for power (Chapter 3) and aerobic and anaerobic fitness (Chapter 4). In addition, our core mus-cles (Chapter 5) are engaged as stabilizers and our balance (Chap-ter 6) is improved through the demands of controlling an external weight through a full range of motion (Chapter 7). Finally, due to the complexity of the movements, the communication and connection between the mind and body and one's kinesthetic awareness are improved.

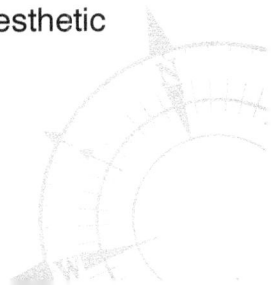

*"Core strenth is critical
to whole-body functional
performance"*

# CHAPTER 5:

## CORE CONDITIONING

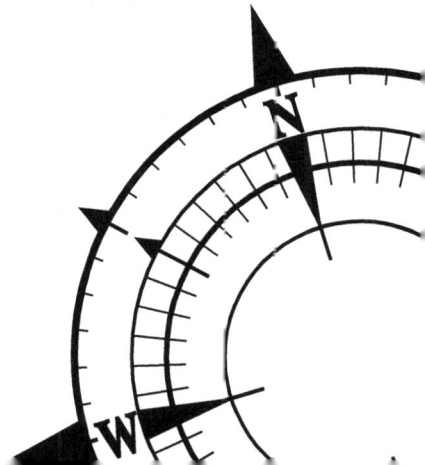

Core strength is critical to the functional performance of any dynamic activity. The core (including the hip flexors, lower back, and abdominals) stabilizes the body throughout any functional movement. This group of muscles is particularly important in movements that involve significant hip rotation (e.g., any sawing motion, splitting wood, stacking hay bales, some swimming strokes), as stabilizers when a portion of the body is largely stationary (e.g., rowing and paddling, standing and casting in a current), or offsetting an external rotational force (e.g. manning a mechanical ice auger or drawing back a bow).

The core also facilitates the safe and efficient transfer of power between the lower and upper body. When conditioned and used properly, the core not only maintains the momentum generated in one part of the body as it transfers this momentum to another part of the body, but adds to it. This is crucial to activities that require coordinated, whole body movements to efficiently drive propulsion (e.g., cross country skiing, climbing into a tree stand, underwater swimming when spear-fishing). Peak performance requires that the body function not as a series of largely independent muscle groups, but rather as one fluid and synergistic entity. One instrument can't harmonize. Trained properly, your body can be a symphony. Core strength is critical to whole-body functional proficiency.

Many of the activities outlined in the previous chapters and the chapters to follow engage and strengthen the core. These movements require the use of the core as a stabilizer and enhance the core's role in transferring momentum. Further, several of the exercises (e.g., squats, push presses) specifically develop the hip flexors' ability to generate power. Below, I have included several exercises that specifically train and increase the capacity of the hip flexors, lower back, and abdominals.

# ANCHORED ADOMINAL RAISES —
## COACHING POINTS

1. Lie on your back and reach overhead gripping an object heavy enough to allow you to smoothly conduct this exercise.

2. Keeping your legs largely straight, raise your legs such that your feet are directly over head using your abdominal muscles and your hip flexors.

3. Slowly lower your legs again until your feet are a few inches off the ground and repeat the movement.

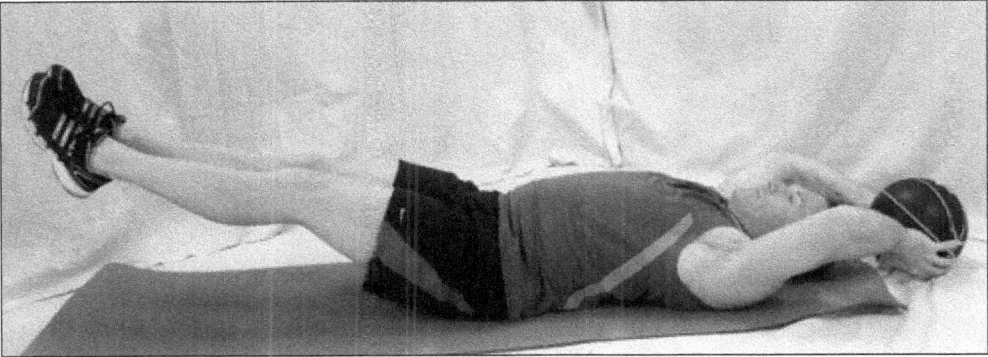

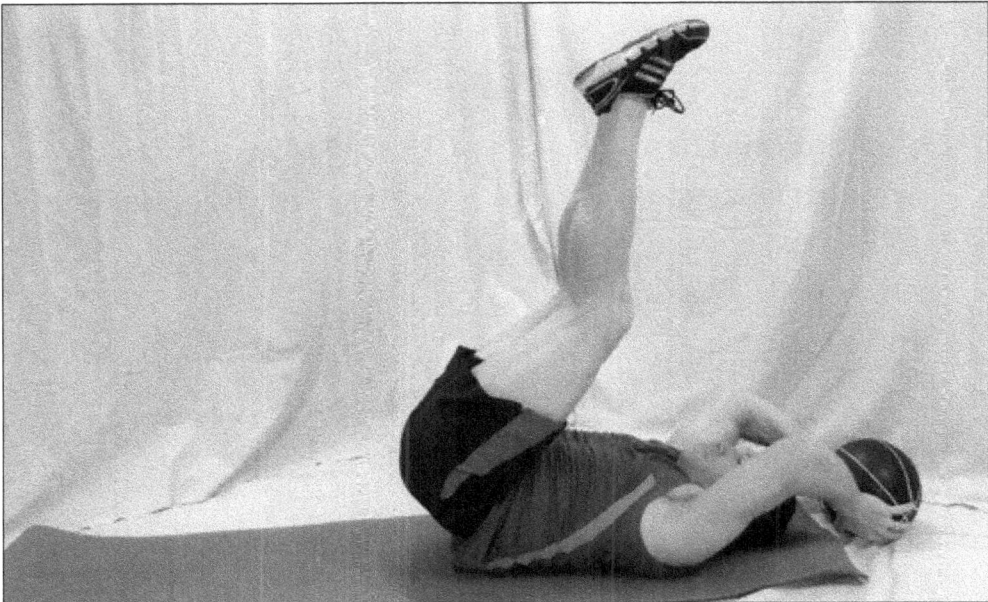

## ABDOMINAL RAISES — COACHING POINTS

1. While hanging from an overhead bar or resting in an abdominal raise chair, allow your legs to hang freely with your toes generally pointed towards the floor.

2. Initiated an upward movement with your abdominals and hip flexors.

3. Bring your knees up towards your chest, pausing for an instant.

4. Slowly lower your legs to your starting position and repeat.

5. You can emphasize either your abdominals by slowing the movement down or your hip flexors by conducting the upward movement in a more explosive manner.

6. You can emphasize your obliques by slightly turning your hips to the side during the entire movement.

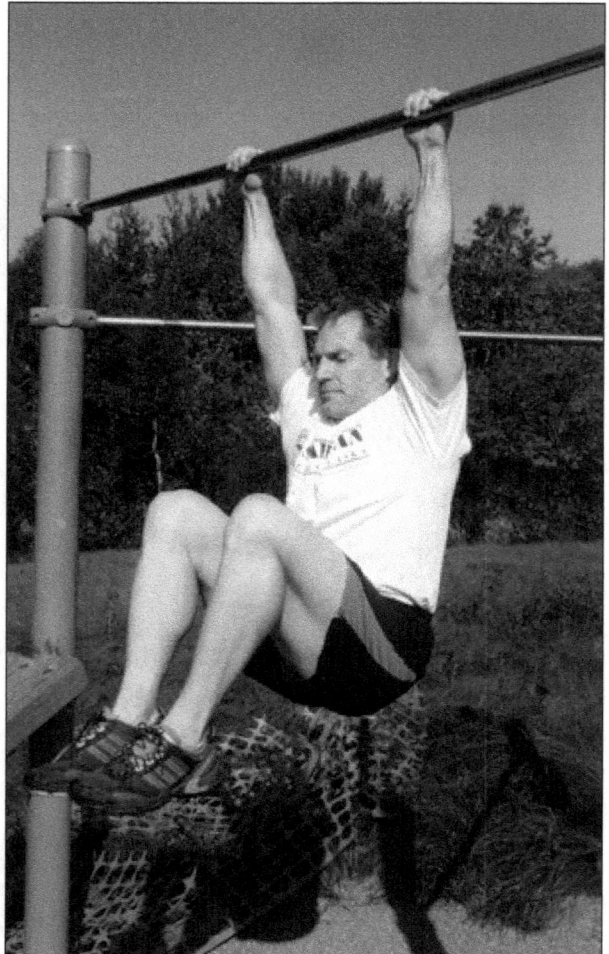

# BICYCLES — COACHING POINTS

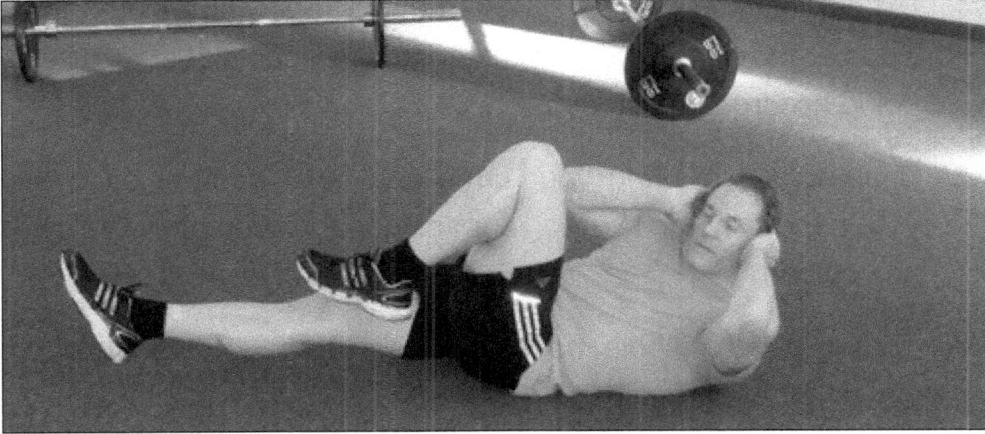

1. Lie on your back and bring your opposite knee and elbow together.

2. Lower both your leg and elbow and then repeat the movement with the other knee and elbow.

3. Throughout the movement, keep both feet and both shoulder blades off the ground.

4. Fully extend and point the toe of the strait leg as the other knee meets the opposite elbow.

5. The head should be resting in your hands. Don't "lift" your head using your hands. The abdominal muscles should do the work.

6. Conduct the entire movement in a slow and controlled manner.

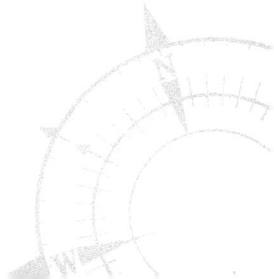

## MOTH TO COCOONS — COACHING POINTS

1. Lie on your back and fully extend your legs with pointed toes. Your arms should be fully extended to your sides. Envision being as large as you can.

2. Simultaneously bring your arms and legs together such that your hands end up next to your ankles. Envision being as small as you can.

3. Throughout the whole movement, keep your feet and shoulders largely off the ground.

4. Conduct the entire movement in a slow and controlled manner.

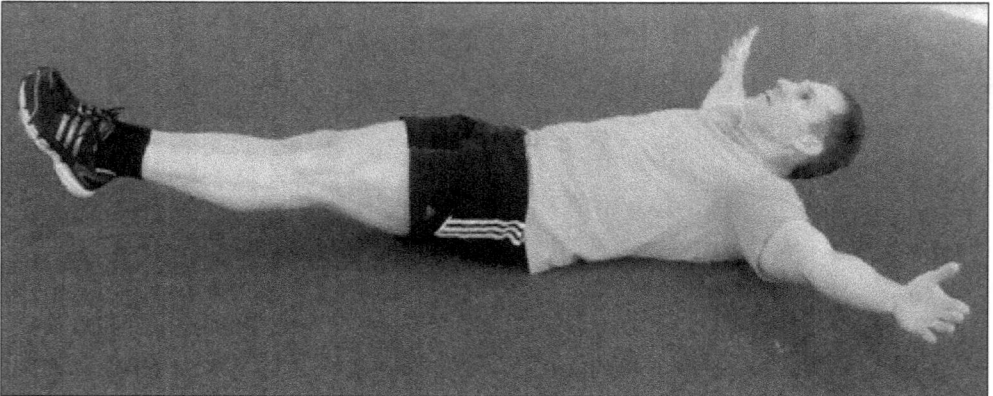

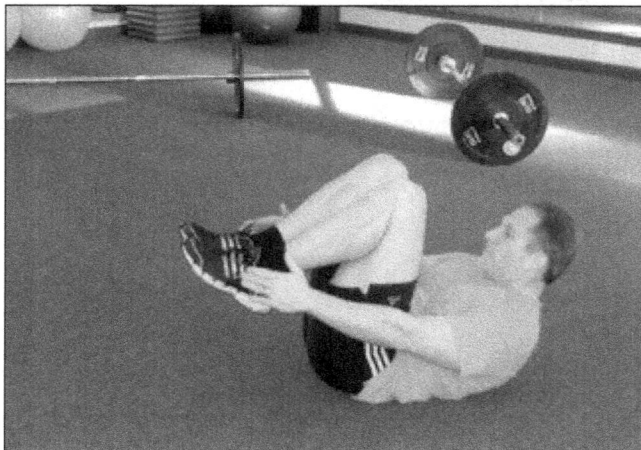

# BIRD DOGS — COACHING POINTS

1. Position yourself on your hands and knees.

2. Raise your opposite arm and opposite leg fully extending both. You want to be as long and straight as you can from the tips of your fingers to the tips of your toes.

3. Hold this position.

4. Return to the starting position and repeat the movement using the other arm and leg.

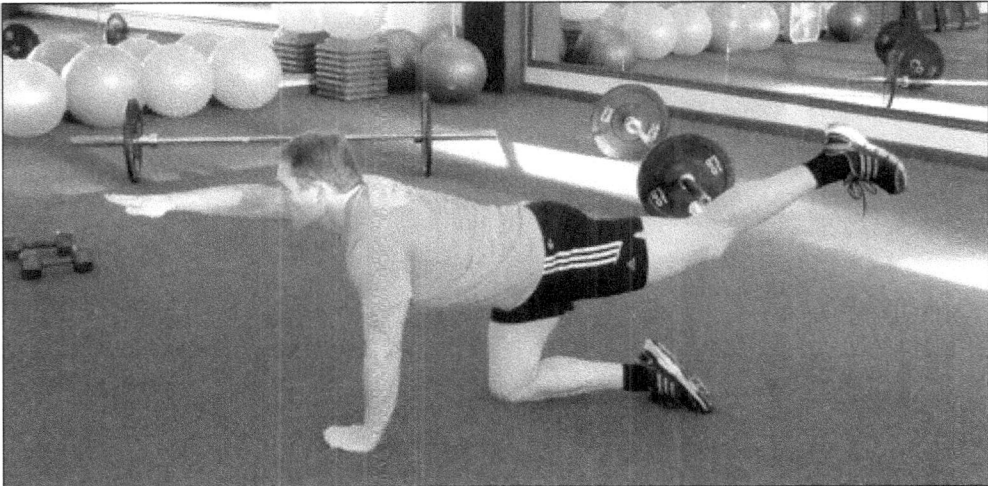

## LYING BACK EXTENSIONS — COACHING POINTS

1. Lie on your stomach and fully extend both arms and both legs.

2. Raise your opposite arm and opposite leg 4-6 inches of the ground.

3. Hold this position.

4. Return to the starting position and repeat with the other arm and leg.

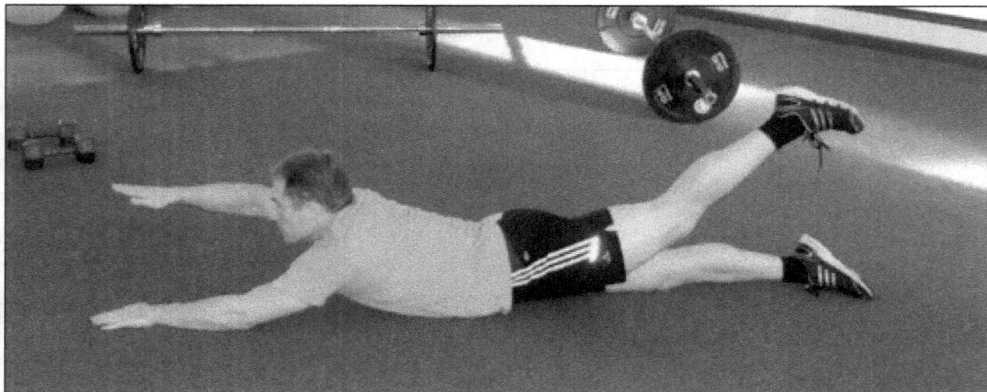

# STRAIGHT LEG DEAD LIFTS —
# COACHING POINTS

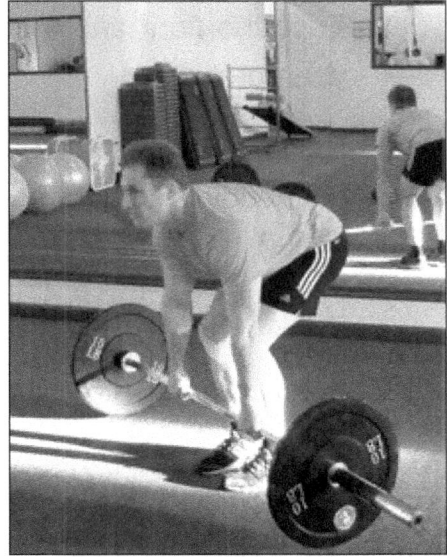

1. Start in a standing position with a slight bend in your knees and holding a bar or object with straight arms. Start with a relatively light weight.

2. Initiate a slight backward movement with the hips and hinge at the waist.

3. Keep your head up, ooking forward throughout the entire movement to maintain a straight back posture.

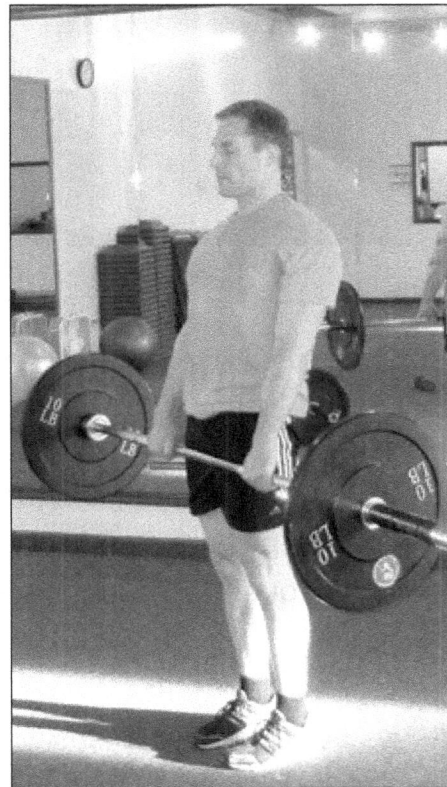

4. Lower yourself until your shoulders are level with or slightly below your waist.

5. Maintaining a rigid back, return to the starting position fully opening your hips.

6. Repeat the movement.

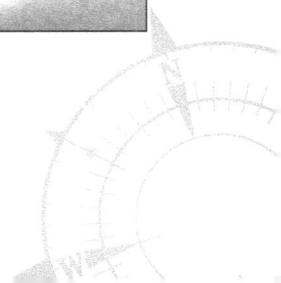

## PLANKS — COACHING POINTS

1. Face the floor and rest on your hands with locked arms or on your forearms.

2. Raise your hips off the floor and maintain rigid posture such that your body is straight from your shoulders to your feet. Your hips should be in line with your body.

3. Hold the position.

4. For increased intensity, raise one leg at a time and hold it.

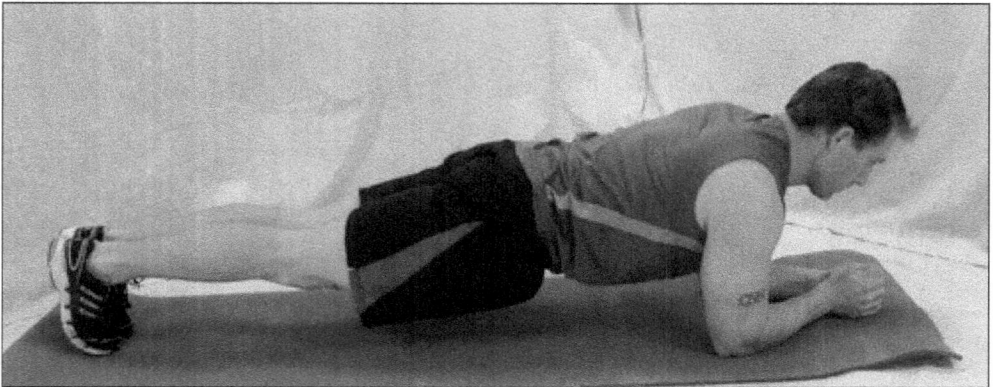

## SIDE PLANKS — COACHING POINTS

1. Face the wall and rest on your forearm or your hand.

2. As with a front plank, raise your hips off the floor and maintain rigid posture such that your body is straight from your shoulders to your feet. Your hips should be in line with your body.

3. Hold the position.

4. For increased intensity, raise your leg and/or your arm.

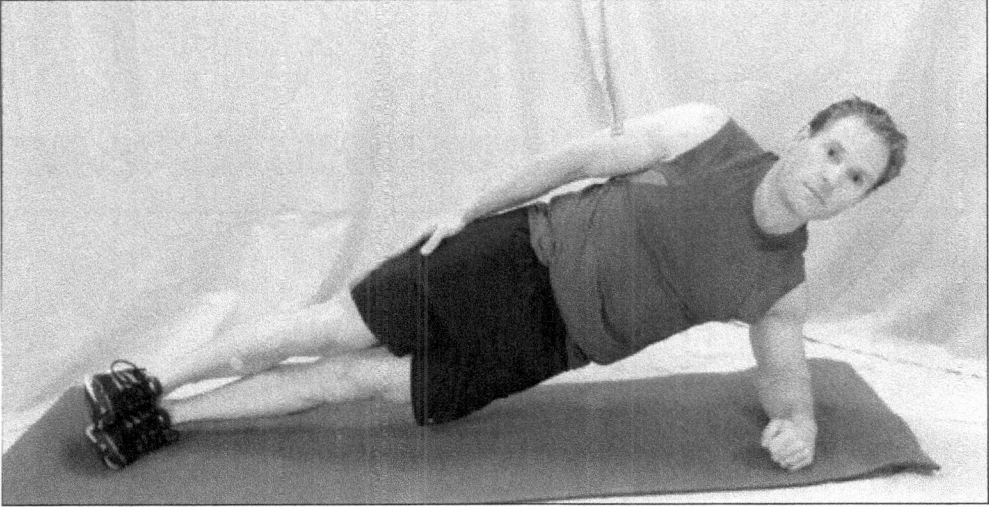

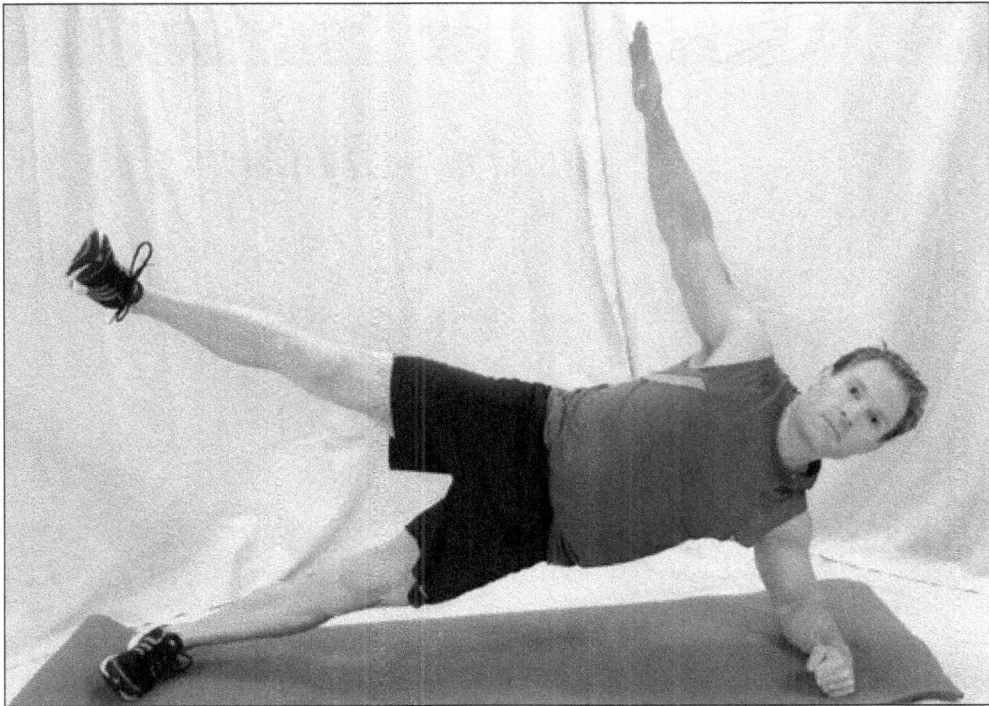

*"Kinesthetic awareness makes you much more capable of dealing with the unexpected"*

# CHAPTER 6:

## BALANCE AND AGILITY

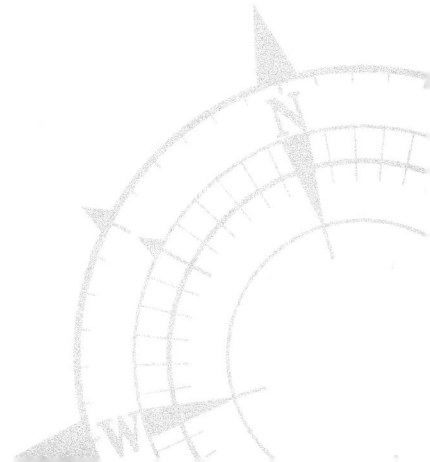

FIT 4 THE FIELD

For many of my clients, the most rapid progress in functional fitness occurs in the areas of coordination, balance, and agility. Improvement is often seen from the first to the second set the first time they perform an exercise.

I postulate that this rapid improvement occurs for three major reasons. The first is that coordination, balance, and agility are woefully under-trained and underdeveloped in most individuals. Many traditionally "fit" individuals don't employ enough activities that benefit these components because the majority of the exercises they use are linear and artificially stabilized (think of the machine circuit at any health club).

The second reason I think rapid improvement occurs is that we all grew up running, skipping, jumping, throwing, and climbing. Playground activities and exploring the woods, streams, and fields all rely on and develop balance, coordination, and agility. The point is that our bodies know how to do these things. At some point, most of us "grew up" and we just stopped doing them. Thus, it is not much of a stretch to challenge our body to relearn some of these skills.

The final reason rapid improvement occurs is that these exercises are fun. Clients love the challenge that comes with balance and agility training.

Functional fitness gains in balance and agility transfer easily and noticeably to everyday activities and recreational endeavors. For those that hunt, fish, and trap, I could make a sound argument that

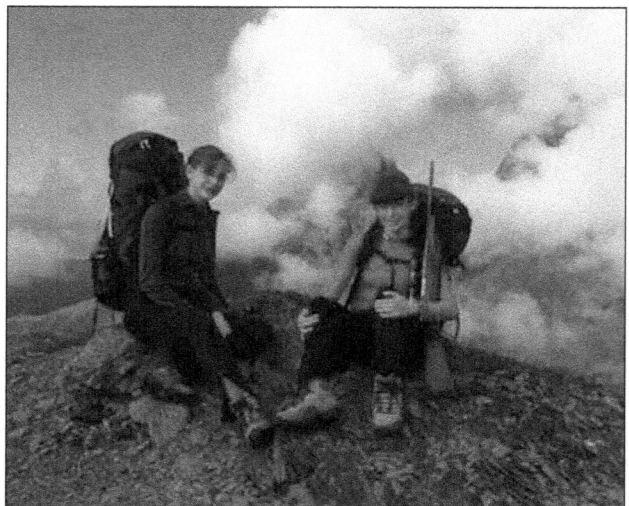

balance and agility are the most important aspects of fitness due to the variable nature of the challenges outdoorsmen face. Climbing in and out of a canoe, mount-ing a horse, traversing the floats of a float plane all rely on balance and agility.

Another very significant result of training the functional fitness components of coordination, balance, and agility is the kinesthetic awareness that you develop. Simply put, you become consciously and subconsciously aware of where your body and its various parts are in relation to each other and the world around you. This gained body awarenessis an almost spiritual revelation to many under-trained individuals and is invaluable in its own right.

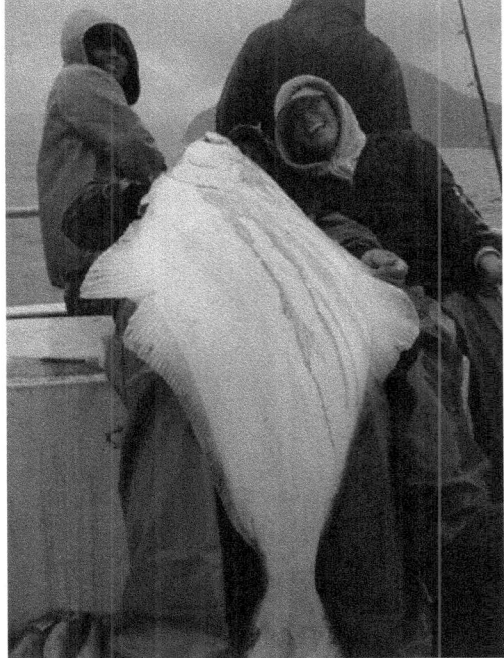

But, of equal significance is that this kinesthetic awareness makes you much more capable of dealing with the unexpected— the algae covered stone in the murky current, the afternoon snow storm that reduces your visibility and ices your footing, the rainstorm and gales that turn your boat deck into a skating rink.... You are better prepared for the surprises life throws at you.

Below are several dynamic exercises that will significantly improve your coordination, balance, and agility.

## SPEED SKATERS

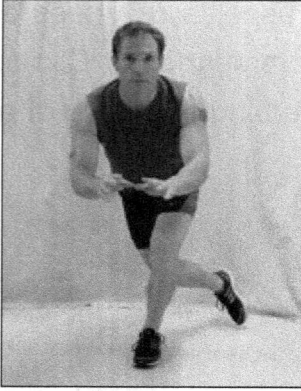

You can perform speed skaters with your body weight or with a medicine ball. Effective, quick, and controlled transfer of body weight from one foot to another, not only in the forward plane but in the lateral plane as well, is a fundamental skill required in virtually any athletic activity.

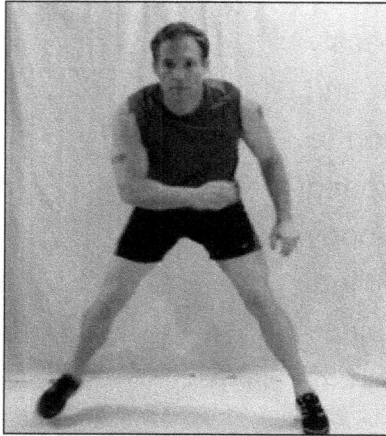

Stride from side to side, emulating the movement seen by speed skaters or skate skiers. You want to keep your head up, your body low, and move athletically. You should challenge yourself by exerting enough effort to allow a broad stride and challenge your balance by spending significant time on one foot and gaining control of the outward momentum you've generated.

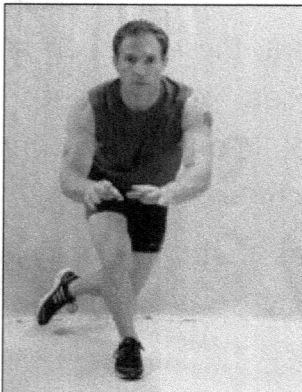

# JUMPS

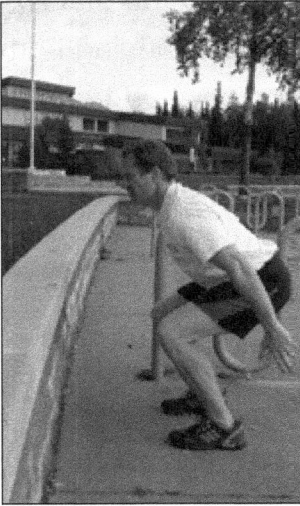

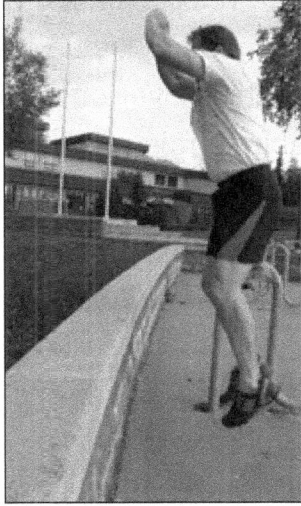

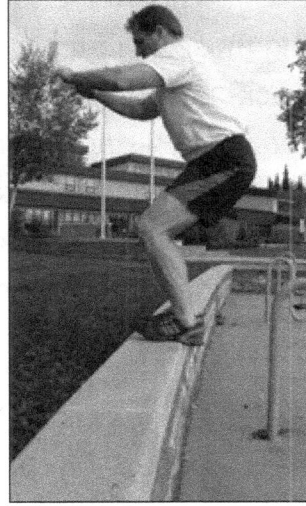

Jumping is a very natural and functional movement that can be performed in a wide variety of ways to develop power, balance, and agility. This activity develops explosive leg strength and power that can be utilized when hiking, climbing, or lifting objects. In addition to the strength developed in the jump, the landing develops balance and coordination. Single leg jumps further these capacities and replicate practical movements like stream crossings.

# SINGLE LEG HOPS

This exercise will develop balance and develop the stabilizing muscles of the lower leg. Many outdoor endeavors ranging from back-country skiing to climbing over obstacles like downed trees or fences to hiking on variable terrain require that your body weight be supported and maintained by a single leg. If you are stable on one foot, you will be rock solid on two feet. Single leg hops should be performed forward and backward as well as side to side.

## FRONT TO BACK

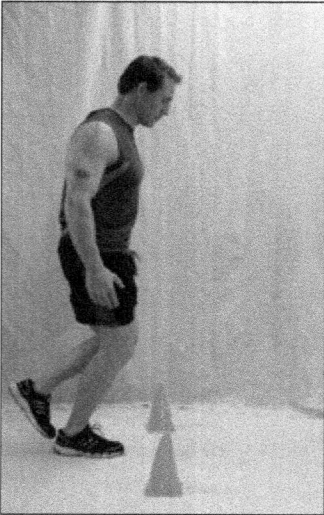
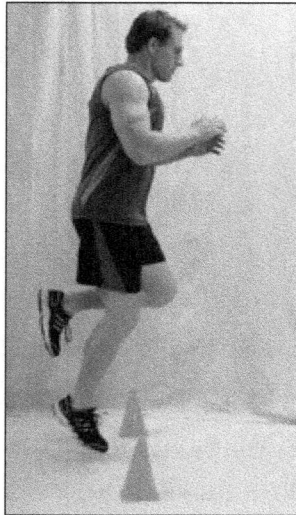
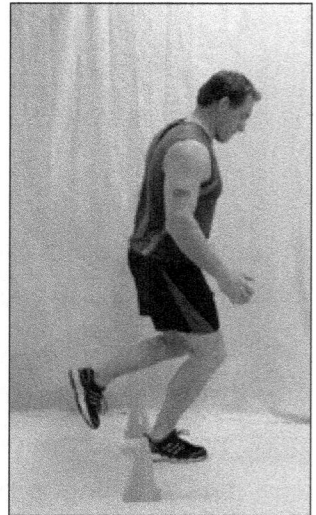

## SIDE TO SIDE

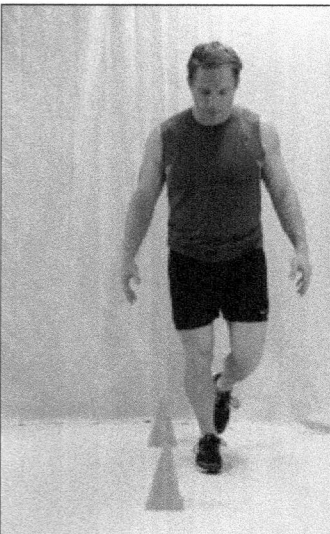
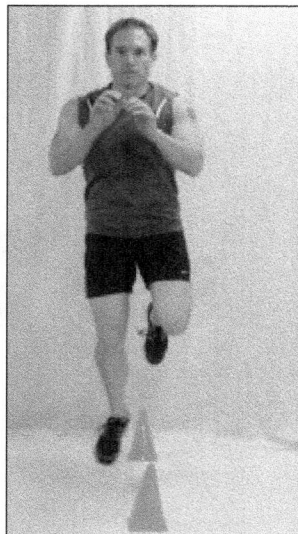
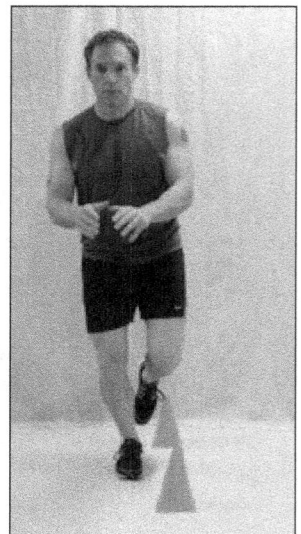

# LEG ABDUCTIONS AND ADDUCTIONS

These exercises enhance balance and strengthen the muscles of the inner and outer thighs, hips, and lower leg. Stand on one leg and raise the other leg to the side and away from your body (abduction) while keeping your knee straight. Similarly, remain standing on the same leg and raise the other leg up and across your body (adduction) as high as possible while keeping your leg straight. The higher you lift your leg, the greater the effort of the hip muscles and challenge to your balance.

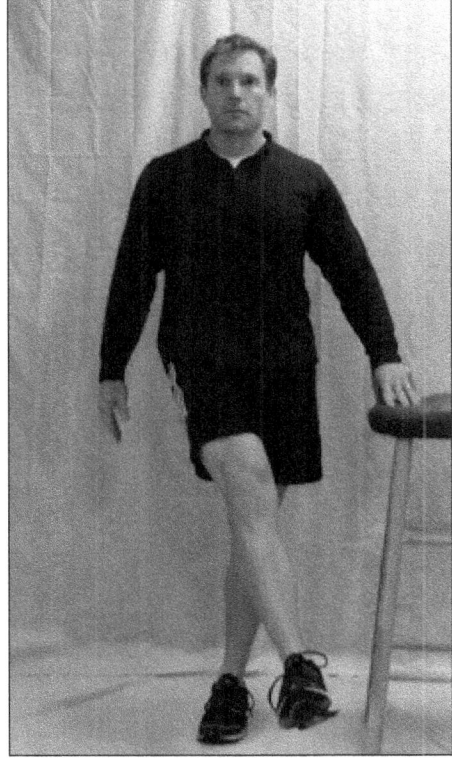

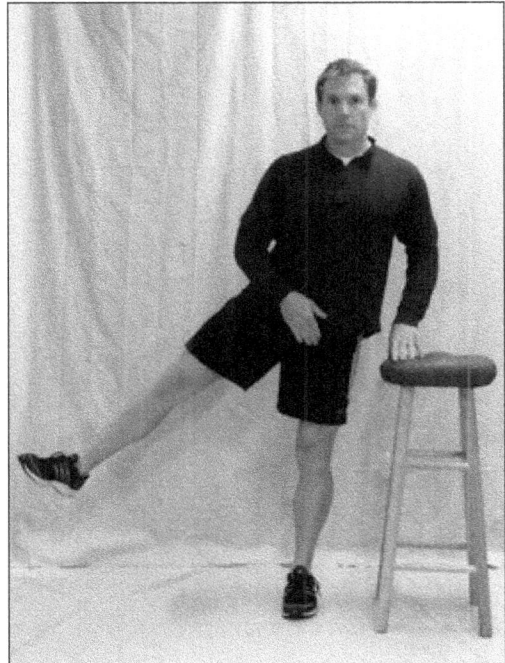

# MEDICINE BALL TOE TAPS

This exercise is very effective at developing quick feet, balance, and coordination. Your goal is to tap the top of the ball with alternate feet as quickly as you can. Start slowly and build up speed as your balance allows. You should keep your eyes on the ball throughout the exercise, as it can roll. The quick foot movement, agility, and accurate foot placement are essential when you travel off-trail, particularly on the descent. In addition to developing agility, medicine ball toe taps require significant oxygen and thus provide metabolic benefit as well.

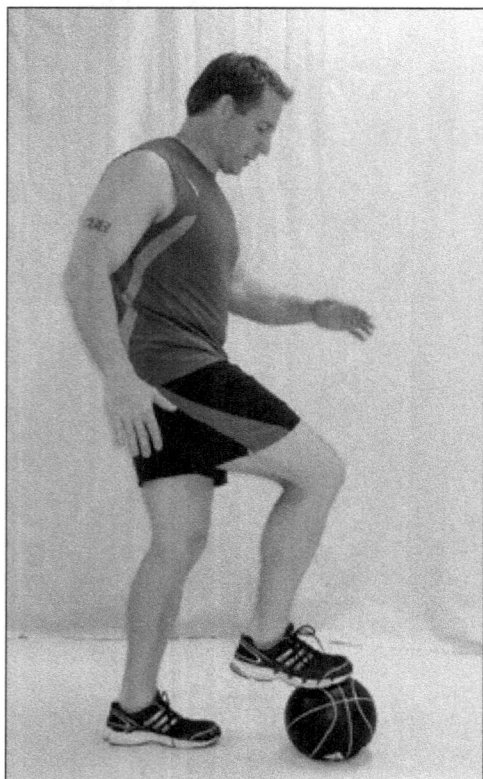

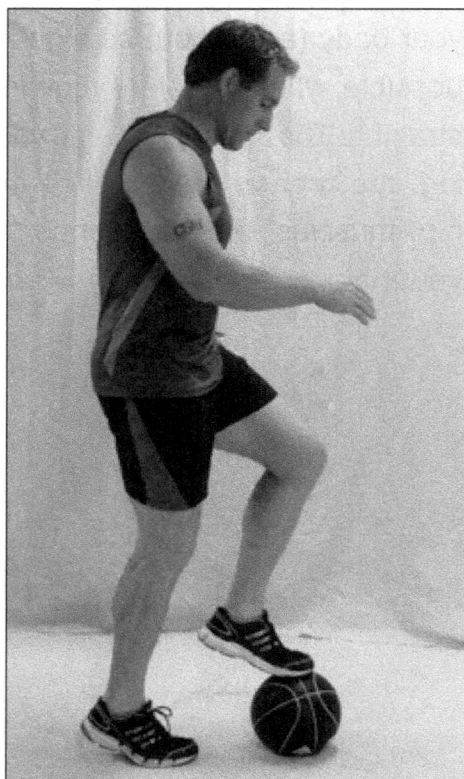

# SWING KICKS

Swing kicks develop coordination by requiring body control in both the forward and lateral planes. Significant time is spent on one leg, thus enhancing balance. Further, the hip flexors are fully engaged throughout the movement. The combination of balance and high stepping has practical applications when crossing streams, climbing over fences, overcoming obstacles such as downed logs and boulders. Hip flexor power and muscular endurance benefit the hip rotation and stabilization utilized in many common activities such as sawing, splitting wood, or standing in a current.

## RIGHT LEG

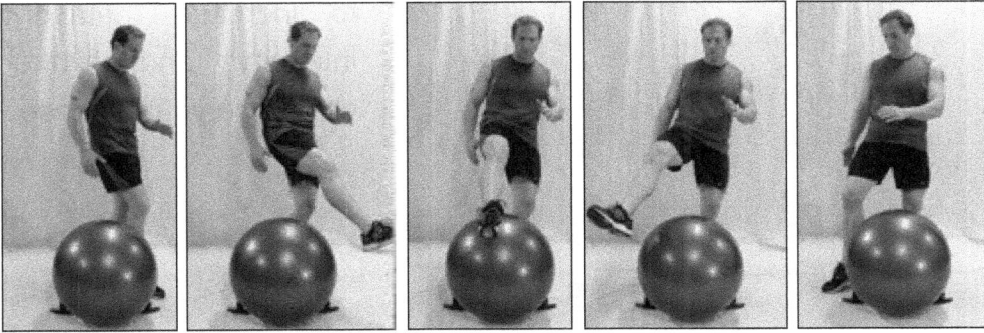

## LEFT LEG

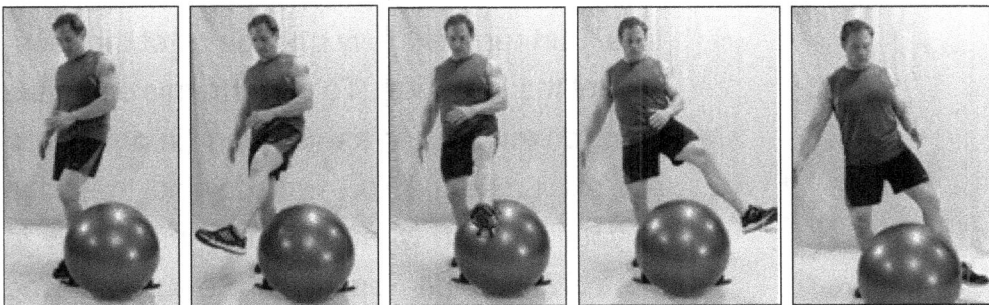

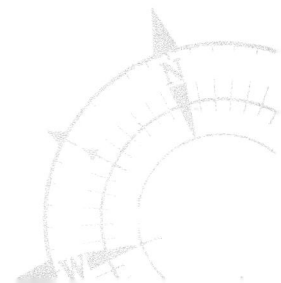

## STEP UPS – FORWARD AND SIDE TO SIDE

Step ups develop foot speed, agility, and coordination. These exercises have obvious applications for activities including hiking and climbing. However, active and agile footwork are critical for other endeavors such as skiing, snow shoeing, and maneuvering on a boat deck. Step ups should be performed forwards and backwards as well as side to side. Increase speed or step height to increase metabolic intensity and further challenge your balance.

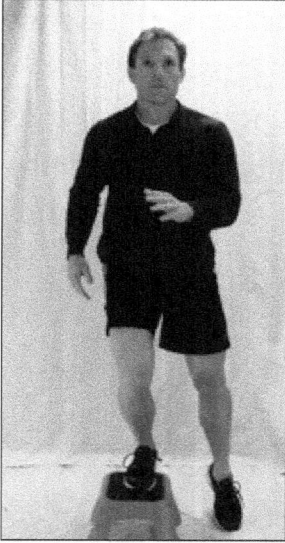

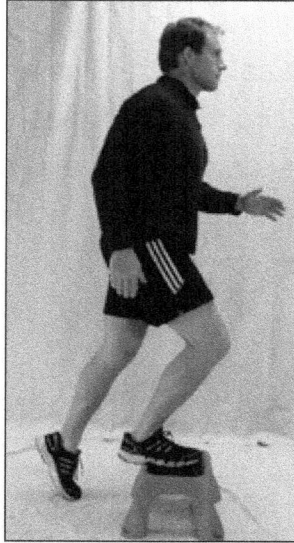

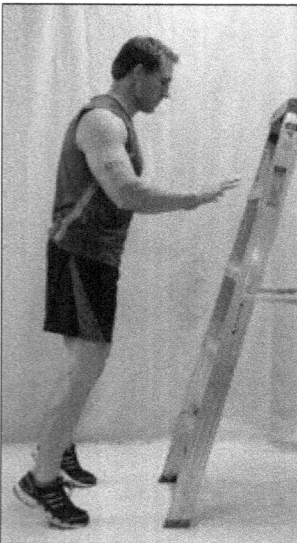

## CALF LEANS

Calf leans enhance your ability to control your body weight in a forward leaning posture. Further, they fully engage all of the muscles of the lower leg. To perform this exercise, lean forward as far as you can (imagine you are ski jumping). You want to find the edge of your balance where you are just barely in control and hold this position. Be sure to stand near a wall or other supportive structure so you can prevent a full fall forward.

# AGILITY RUNS

We want to be proficient not only in the forward plane, but also the lateral plane. Sideways runs and shuffles engage the lateral muscles of the upper thigh and the muscles of the lower leg. This has practical benefits for any activity that involves moving over variable terrain or utilizes significant lateral movement. In addition, this activity enhances agility and coordination. When performing these exercises, keep your head up, your bottom down, and your feet quick.

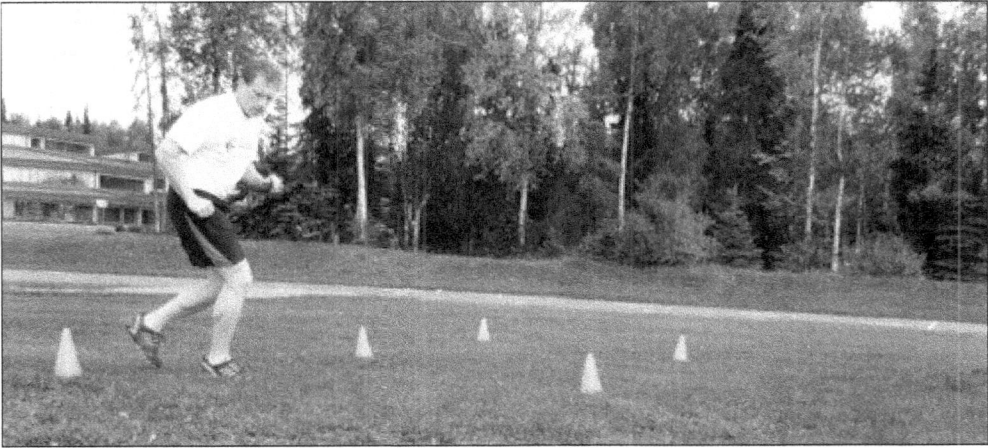

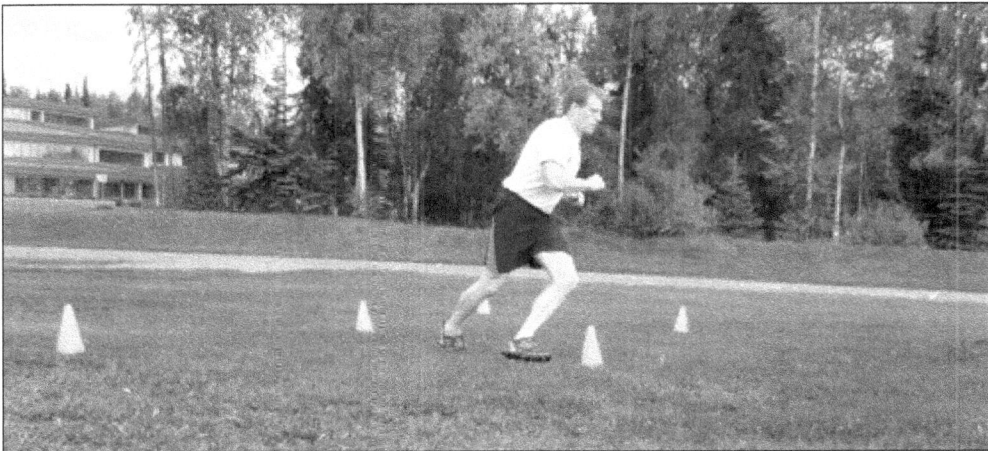

## MEDICINE BALL WALL TOSSES

Medicine ball wall tosses are simply a thruster where the ball is launched upward and then caught as it returns earthward. Similar to thrusters, this exercise enhances one's ability to generate and transfer power from the legs to the upper body and overhead. Medicine ball wall tosses also challenge one's focus and coordination.

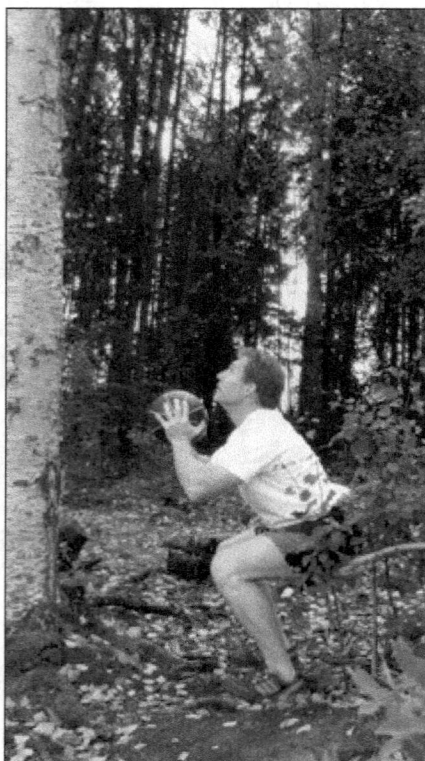

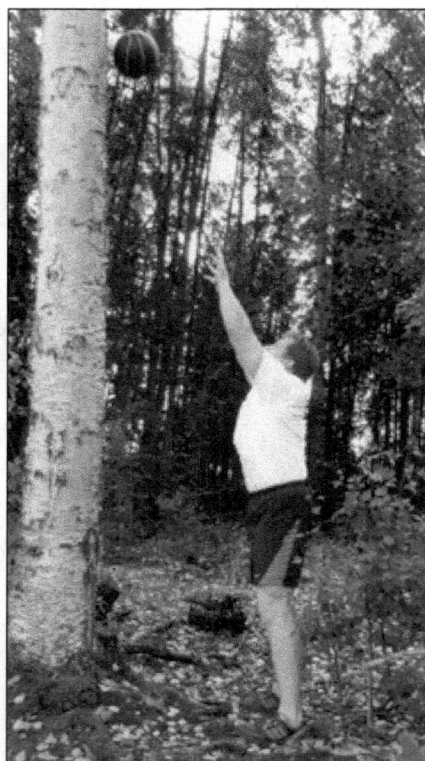

## ROPE AND WALL CLIMBING

Climbing, when performed correctly, is an outstanding full-body movement that requires significant coordination. Ensure that your climbing environment is safe.

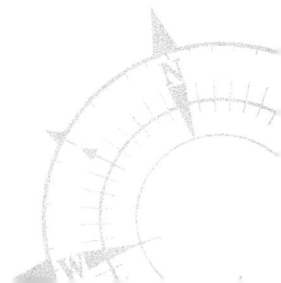

*"You can produce more power by moving your muscles and joints through their full range of motion"*

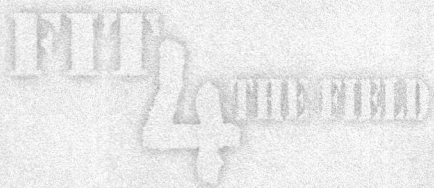

# CHAPTER 7:

## FLEXIBILITY

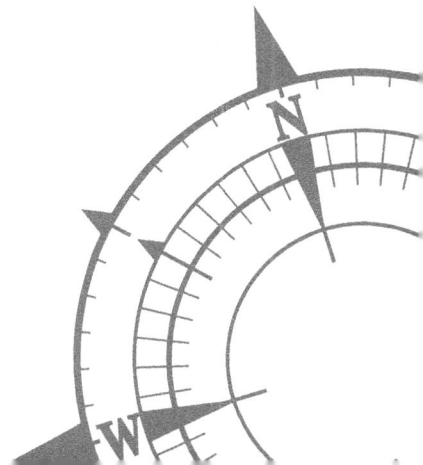

Flexibility is the elasticity of an individual muscle group (e.g., the hamstrings) and range of motion is the multiplanar movement potential across a joint. These two components of fitness are critical to all aspects of physical performance. Similar to balance and agility, these aspects are often significantly under-trained. The benefits of increased flexibility and range of motion are twofold. The first is that risk of injury is reduced when you encounter activities at the edge of your abilities. The second is that you can produce more power by moving your muscles and joints through their full range of motion. Utilizing the full range of motion across joints is like opening the throttle of an engine. The net result is greater energy and power delivery. This principle applies to any physical activity. Significant performance improvements can be gained by fully utilizing the mechanical advantages available from the hips, hamstrings, and shoulder girdle.

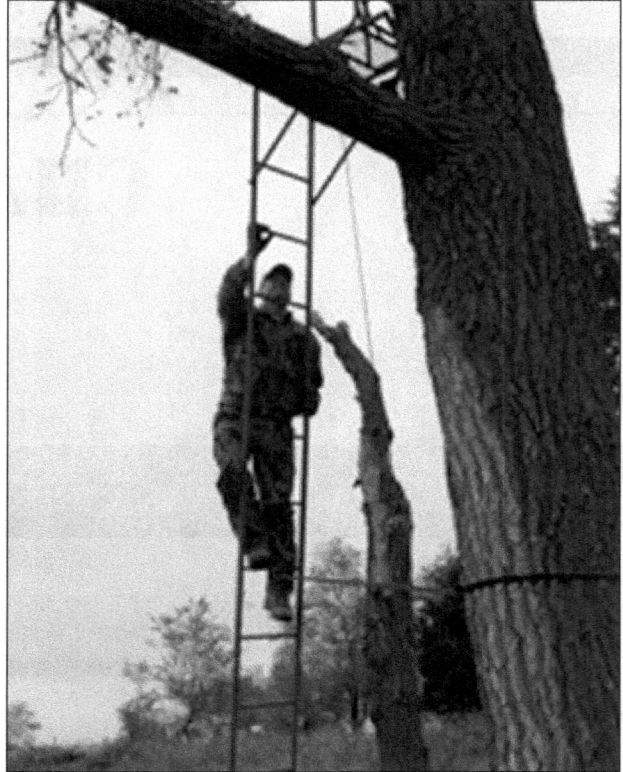

There are two primary and complementary ways that flexibility and range of motion can be dramatically improved. The first is performing all of the activities described in previous chapters through their full range of motion. As one example, it is generally not advisable to do deep squats (i.e., where the hips drop well below the level of the knee) with an external load. However, body weight or light weight squats can be done as deep as your body allows. Range of motion will improve with practice through time. Recognize that billions of humans throughout the world eat, pray, converse, and relieve themselves in a deep squat, even at advanced ages.

The second way to improve flexibility and range of motion is through deliberate stretching exercises. There are dozens of stretches one can perform to improve flexibility and range of motion. Further, certain forms of exercise include a primary focus on these fitness components (e.g., yoga, Pilates). I recommend including stretching in your warm up to reduce the risk of pulls or strains. During the warm up phase of your workout, hold

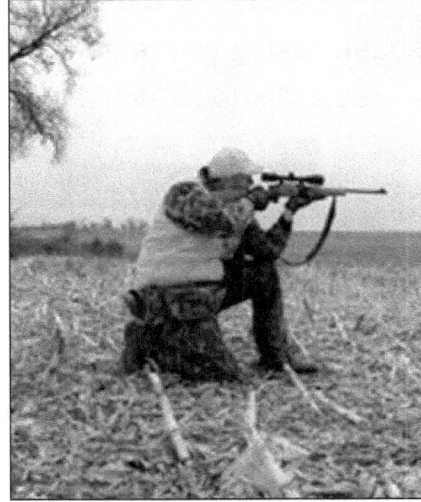

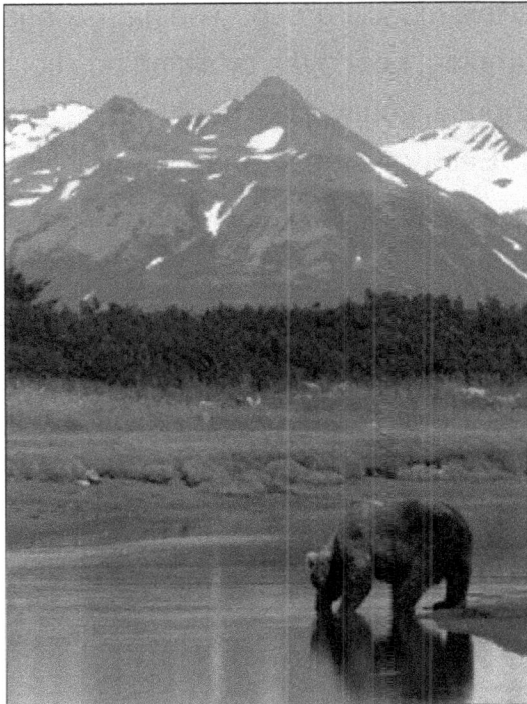

each stretch for 10-15 seconds. At the end of your workout, stretch again. Because your body temperature is elevated, this is a good time to increase your flexibility and range of motion. At the end of your workout, I recommend holding each stretch for at least 30 seconds. Below are a few basic stretches that address the primary muscle groups and joints of the body.

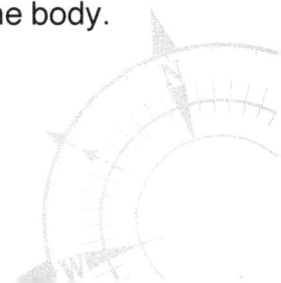

# GROIN AND INNER THIGH

To stretch the groin and inner thigh, drop into a wide, deep squat. Using your elbows for leverage, slowly and gently open your knees wider to stretch the inner thigh.

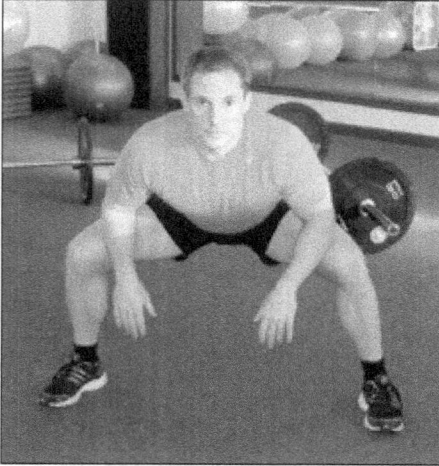

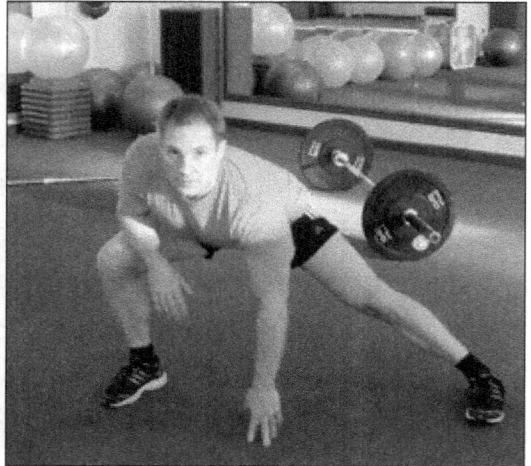

# HAMSTRINGS

Tight hamstrings are common in many individuals. Thus, particular attention should be paid to this muscle group. The hamstrings can be stretched in an upright standing, bent over, or sitting position. Regardless of the position you choose, you want to gently place and hold tension on the hamstrings. Each of these variations will also stretch the lower back.

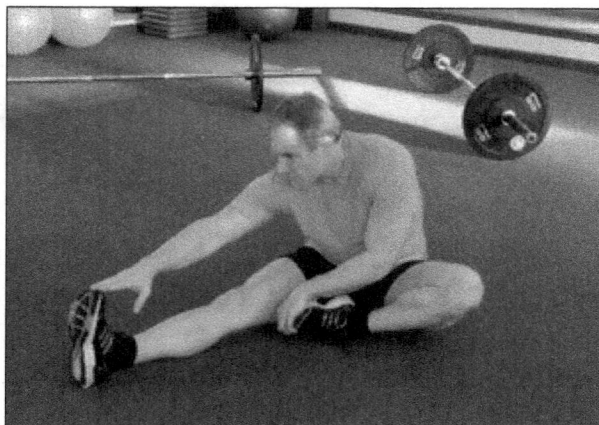

## HIP FLEXORS

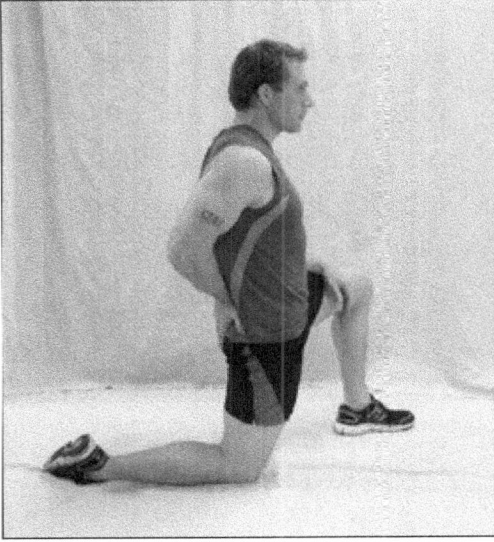

To stretch the hip flexors, kneel on one knee and roll your hips forward. You can aid this stretch by pushing on your rump from behind.

## QUADRICEPS

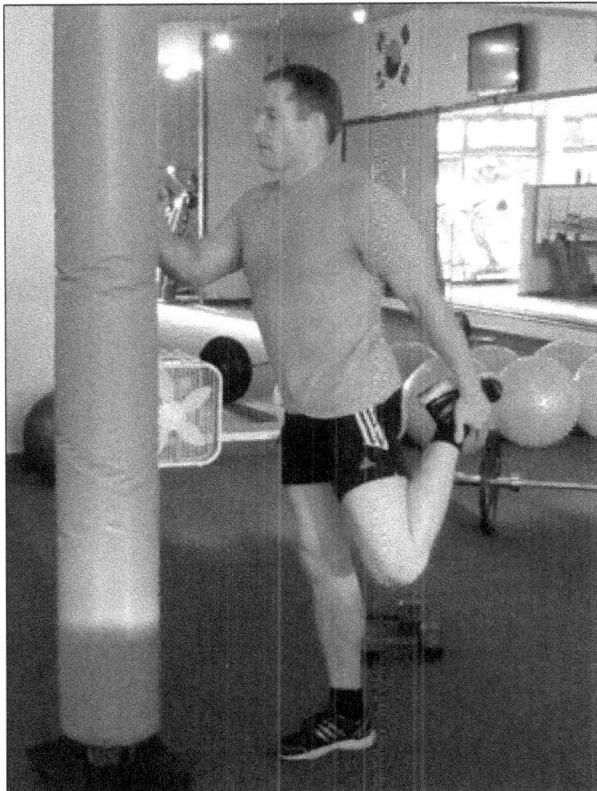

The quadriceps are best stretched from a standing position. Grasp the front of your foot just below the ankle and slowly and gently apply force to stretch the quadriceps muscle group. Ensure you have a wall or other object available to assist your balance.

## CALVES

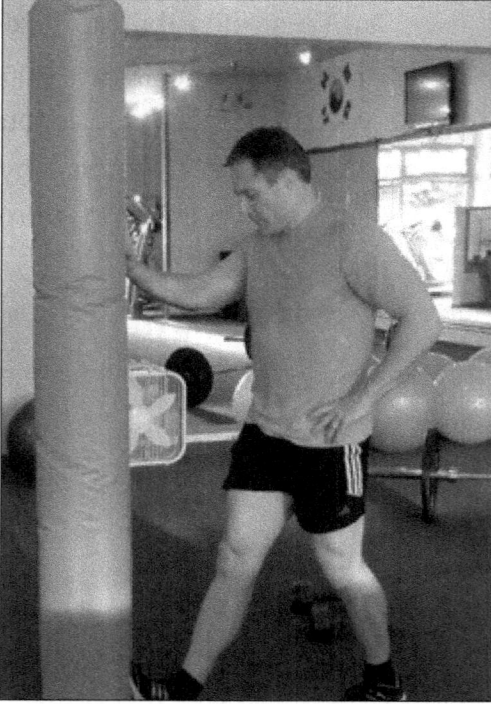

The calves can be stretched by placing your toes against a wall and heel on the floor forming a roughly 45° angle between your foot and the floor. Keeping your leg straight, slowly press your body towards the wall with your other foot and leg.

## SHOULDERS

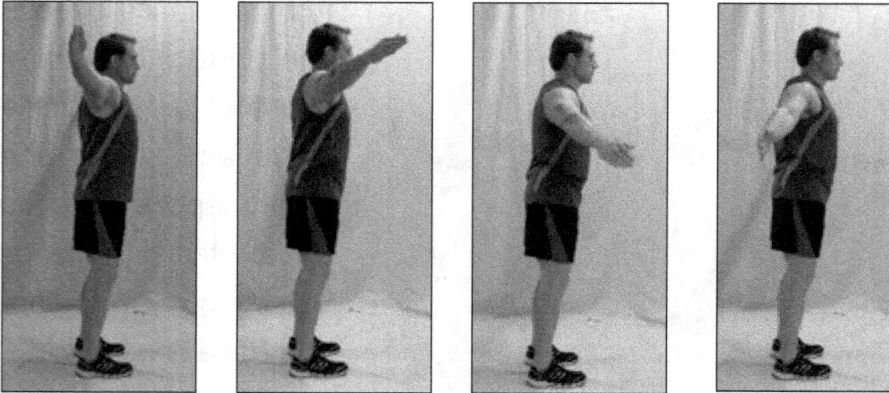

To improve flexibility in the shoulder girdle, hold your arms directly away from your body as if forming the shape of a cross. Begin rotating your arms forward forming small circles with your hands and slowly increase the size of the circle until you are at your full range of motion in the shoulder joint. Repeat this movement, but in the reverse direction.

# CHEST

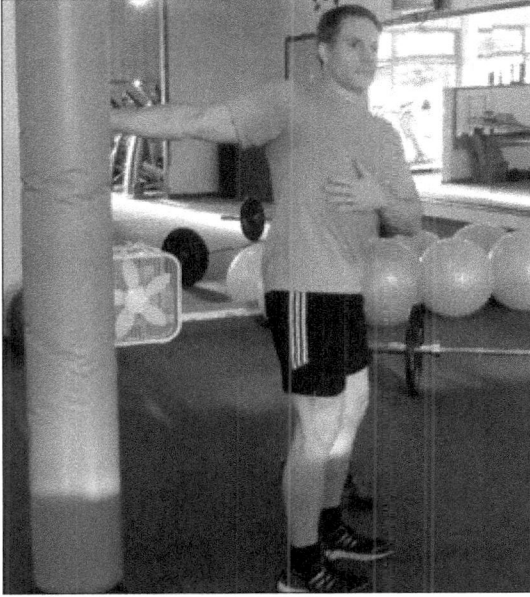

The chest can be stretched effectively by placing your hand on a static object such as a pole or wall. Simply rotate your body away from this object to open your chest and your body weight will provide the force producing the stretch.

# BACK

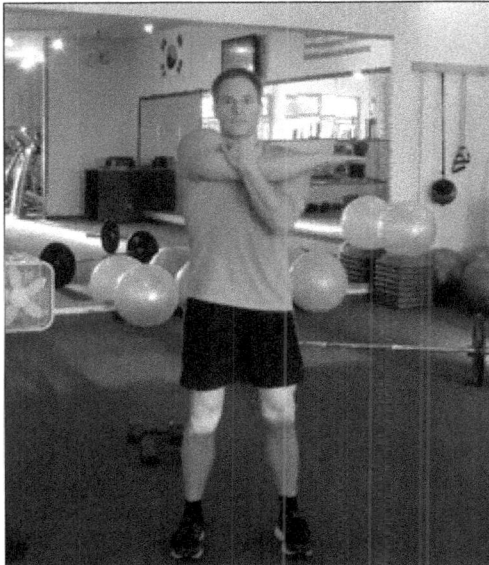

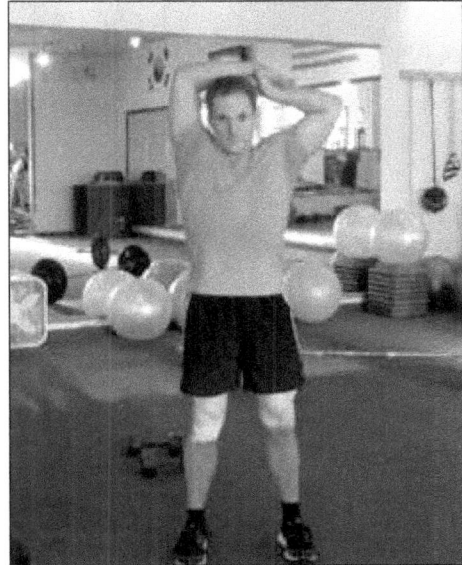

To stretch your back, use the leverage available in your arms by pulling each arm across and above your body. Also, interlock your fingers and reach fully over head to stretch your spinal muscles.

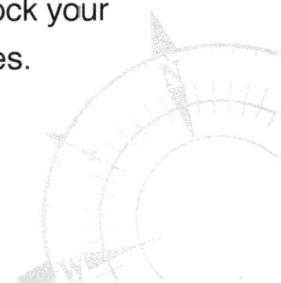

# NECK

To warm up and stretch the neck, simply roll your head slowly and deliberately several times clockwise. Repeat the movement in the opposite direction.

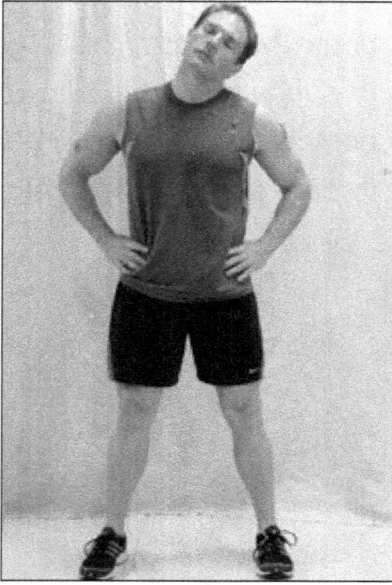

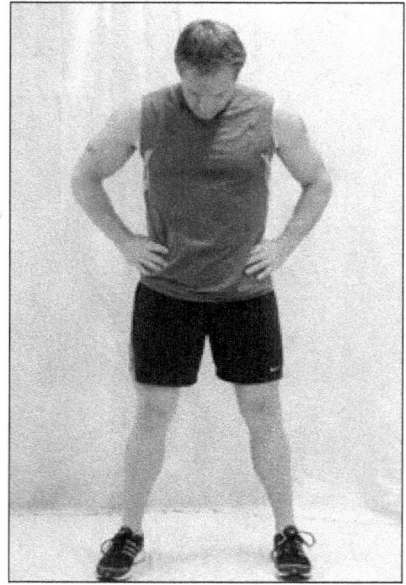

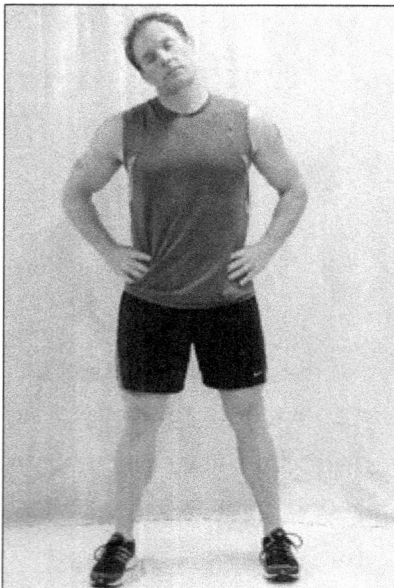

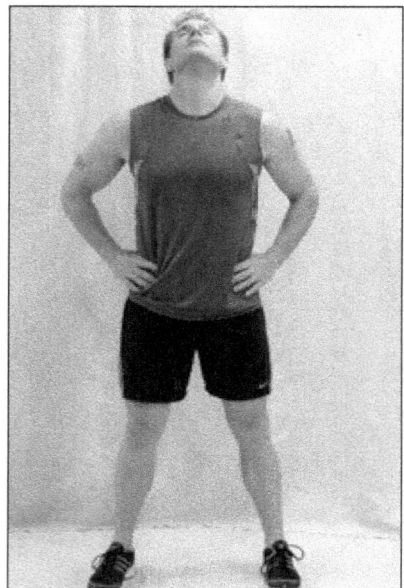

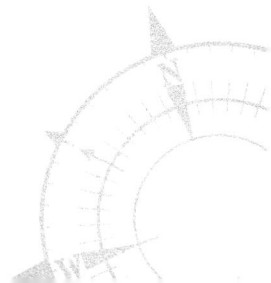

*"Engaging in new activites challenges your fitness in novel ways"*

# CHAPTER 8:

## RECREATION AS TRAINING

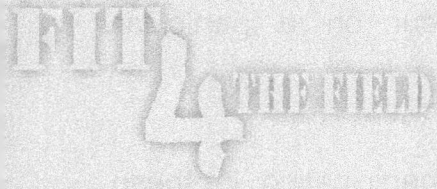

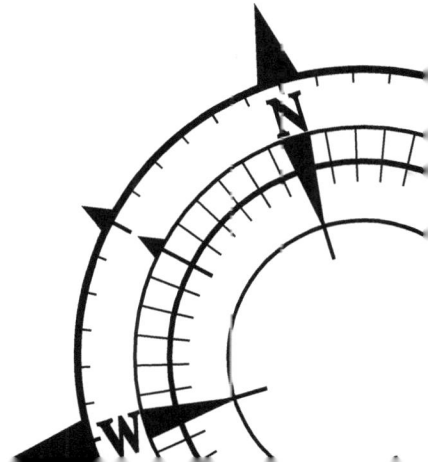

FIT 4 THE FIELD

Running, biking, swimming, hiking, climbing, skiing, snow-shoeing, canoeing, and kayaking can all provide multiple benefits across the fitness components addressed in the preceding chapters. As functional movements, they inherently benefit functional fitness. These enjoyable activities can provide diversity, both physical and mental, to workout programming, and the practice of a variety of activities allows you to train throughout the year regardless of the climate you live in. They can be part of pre-season scouting for hunters and trappers as they learn the lay of the land to gain insights into where different species occur on a particular landscape.

While there is obvious benefit to participating in these activities purely for their enjoyment, a different mindset is needed when engaging in these pursuits as part of a program with the intent of improving overall performance.

Include variation in your program not only by perform-ing multiple activities such as biking, running, rowing, and swimming, but by varying your approach within a specific activity. For exam-ple, conduct long, relatively slow hikes or runs on trails with vary-ing terrain that includes uphill and downhill segments and vary the external weight you carry in your pack. It is beneficial to focus on goals of either time or distance in long dura-tion, low intensity sessions. Balance these sessions with other sessions that include shorter dura-tion, higher speed segments (e.g., 400

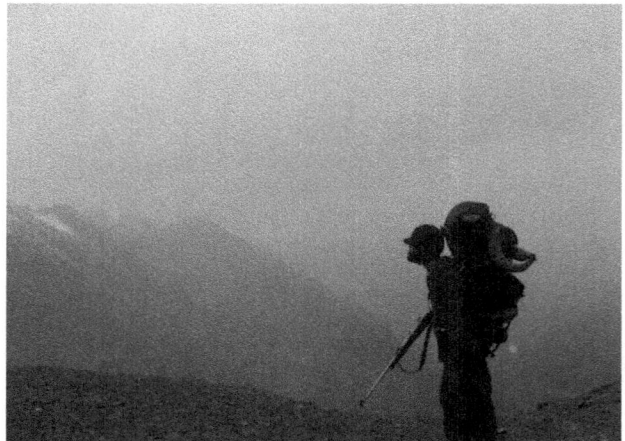

m sprints conducted in a circuit with pushups and medicine ball cleans). Further, you can instill variation within a given session of a given activity. When running along a road, walk from the first light pole to the second, jog to the third, sprint to the fourth, and repeat. Alternatively, walk for a minute, jog for a minute, and run for a minute, and repeat. In essence, we are including periodization and interval training across and within workouts, respectively.

To ensure intensity, monitor your heart rate and time. Watches or wrist bands that include both a timer and a heart rate monitor can be purchased at most sporting goods stores. Timing your activities will provide an accurate assessment of your progression from week to week and month to month. In addition, competing with the clock naturally motivates most individuals.

Below is a chart identifying target heart rates for individuals by age. As previously mentioned, ensure you have consulted with your physician and that these targets are appropriate for you.

| Age *(years)* | Target Heart Rate* *(beats per minute)* |
|---|---|
| <20 | 100-170 |
| 25 | 98-166 |
| 30 | 95-162 |
| 35 | 93-157 |
| 40 | 90-153 |
| 45 | 88-149 |
| 50 | 85-145 |
| 55 | 83-140 |
| 60 | 80-136 |
| 65 | 78-132 |
| >70 | 75-128 |

*range from 50% to 85% of maximum heart rate

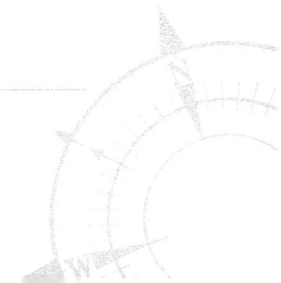

By monitoring both time and heart rate during the course of your activities, you will stay mentally engaged. One of the problems with running on the treadmill at the gym is that many folks are lulled by the television or other distractions. They end up going through the motions. While any physical activity has benefits, distracted efforts minimize gains, reduce efficiency, and dampen the mind-body connection we are striving for.

Look to learn new activities. This will allow you to be active throughout the year and the benefits of developing new skills and training new motor pathways will further utilize and enhance your kinesthetic awareness.

Engaging in new activities will challenge your fitness in novel ways and require a heightened coordination between your mind and your body. Thus, look for new activities to try and seek guidance from enthusiastic experts who enjoy teaching. Don't be bashful about finding a trainer or coach, or joining a class or club (e.g., Nordic ski club, crew team, orienteering group, or trail running association). These activities can then serve as a source of year-round recreational

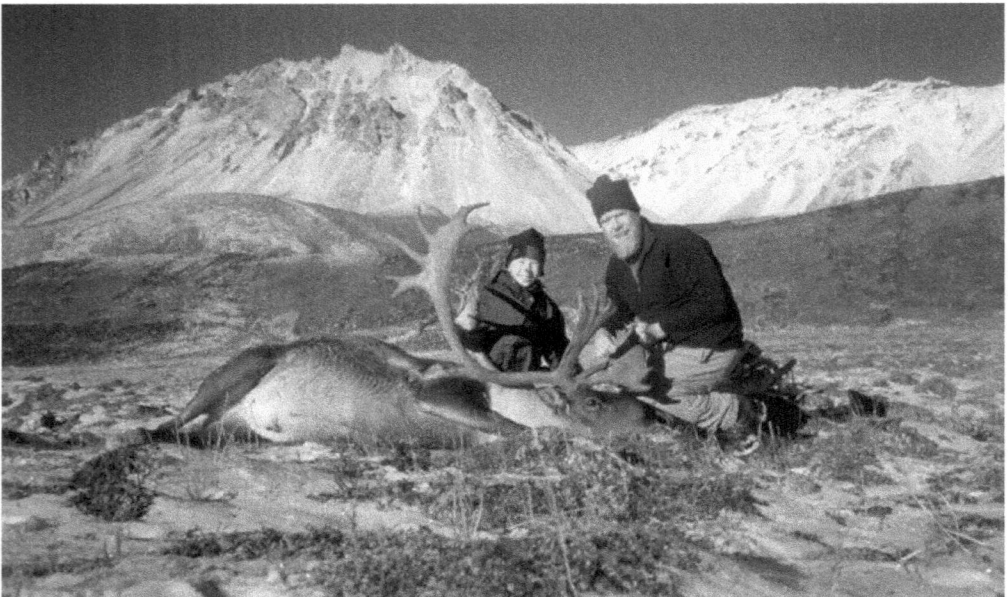

enjoyment and offer new and challenging training opportunities.

For sportsmen, training outside in the environment of their favorite pursuit will be more natural and meaningful. There may be opportunities for training sessions combined with pre-season preparations, such as duck blind maintenance, or civic duties like river clean-ups. When you head outdoors, ensure that you take the same precautions you do when fishing or hunting. Use sun screen and/or fabrics that offer UV protection. Utilize insect repellent and carry bear spray if training in bear country. Know local plants and animals and their habits and behavior. Ensure that your clothing is appropriate for the weather conditions. Carry extra food and water on long training sessions and carry navigation and communication tools and know how to use them. Also, let someone know where you are going and when you expect to return. Appropriate footwear is paramount as is training in first aid. Finally, if you plan to train on snowy slopes, take an avalanche safety course.

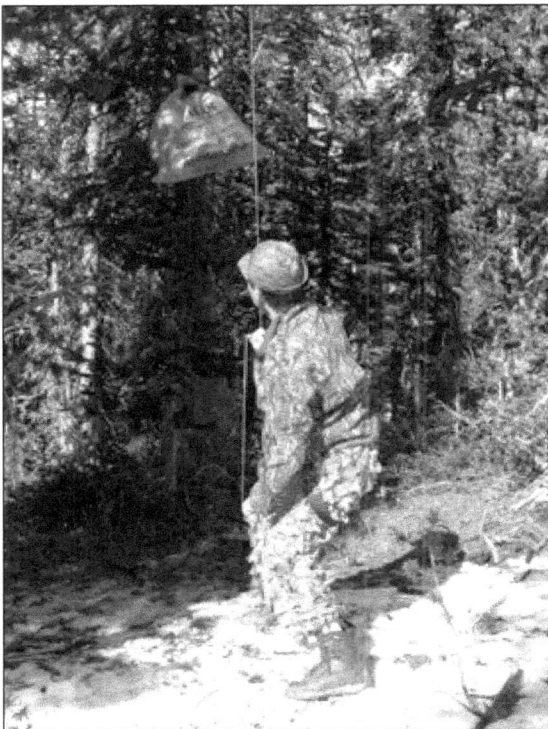

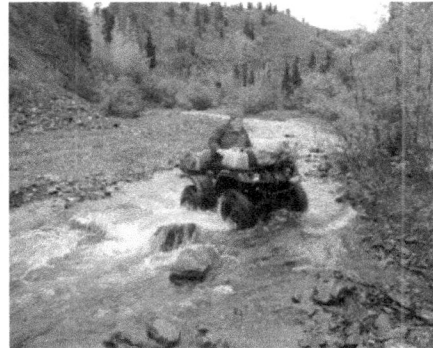

*"Programming is how we turn a stack of rough cut timbers into a tight and sturdy cabin"*

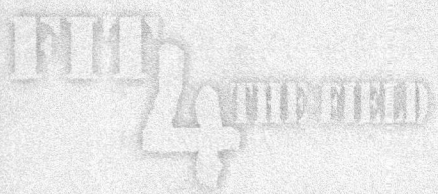

# CHAPTER 9:

## PROGRAMMING

Programming is how we assemble all of the pieces described in the previous chapters. It is how we developed a truly integrated fitness that forms our mosaic of power, endurance, core strength, flexibility, and kinesthetic awareness. It is how we turn a stack of rough-cut timbers into a tight and sturdy cabin.

Programming is part art and part science. The one message I want to convey is that "routine" is to be avoided. Many exercise programs consist of dedicating specific days to specific body parts. For example, one of the classic routines is weight training for the chest, shoulders and triceps on Mondays and Thursdays and back, biceps, and legs on Tuesdays and Fridays. Additional 30-60 minute sessions on a treadmill, elliptical, or stationary bike likely follow the resistance work. Almost all of us who have spent any time in the gym have used some variation of the above program.

Not only were our metabolic pathways (i.e., aerobic and anaerobic) and fitness components (muscular strength and cardiovascular endurance) compartmentalized and trained separately, even our individual muscle groups were further divided, treated so independently that we worked them on separate days. How can this be the best approach to developing functional fitness across a variety of activities in a wide range of environments? It is not an organic approach.

I don't want to imply that all of one's time training in this manner is wasted. In fact, this approach

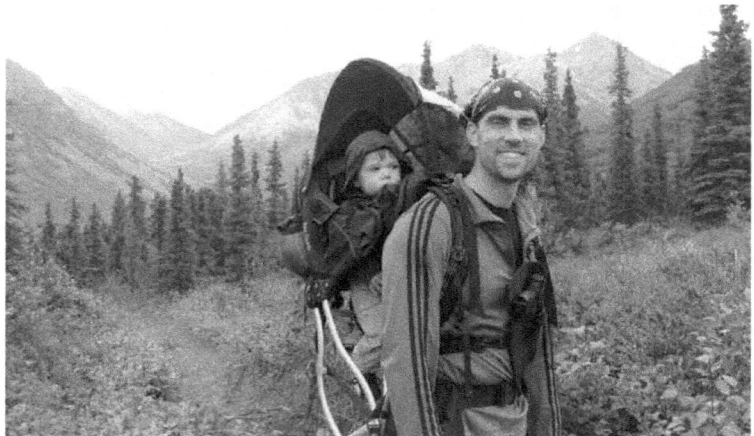

does provide a significant foundation of strength and cardiovascular endurance. However, we can increase the efficiency of our efforts and develop a fitness that s more transferable to the world outside the gym.

Rather, what we should strive for is constant variation in exercises, order, intensity, and execution. We also should structure workout sessions that emphasize both balance and unpredictability. Developing skills in a variety of seasonal activities will allow you to include recreation as part of your training program throughout the year. This approach will consistently stimulate your body to adapt and increase the fitness components discussed in previous chapters. Further, it will avoid the mental boredom and fatigue that comes with over-structured and repeated routines. Finally, the varied approach will lead to a high level of year around functional fitness that will translate well to the variety of physical activities in which you, as an outdoorsman, joyfully participate.

As an example, I have provided a six week program below. Should you chose to follow this regimen, I know that it will serve you well. However, it is simply one example and not a singular routine to be followed in perpetuity. My intent is to illustrate the blending of the different fitness components and the variation that occurs from one workout to the next. Ultimately, I want you to have the knowledge and understanding to take ownership of your own programming and tailor your approach to your specific needs and interests.

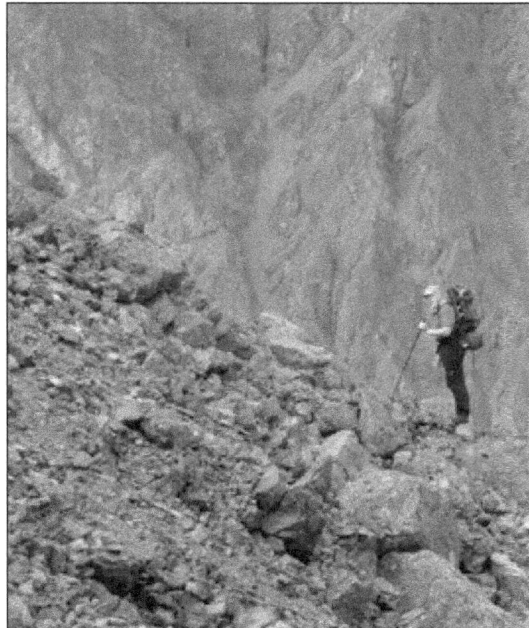

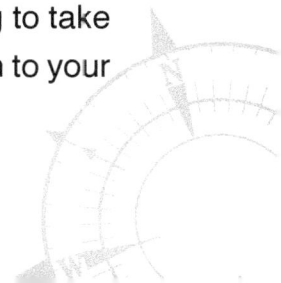

# WEEK 1:

**Day 1 (date):** _____

Five minute warm-up on treadmill, elliptical, bike, rowing machine, etc.

General stretching

| Resistance exercise circuit: | Set 1 | Set 2 | Set 3 | Set 4 |
|---|---|---|---|---|
| Squats (weight/reps) | ___/___ | ___/___ | ___/___ | ___/___ |
| Pull ups/lat pull downs | ___/___ | ___/___ | ___/___ | ___/___ |
| Push ups (reps) | ___ | ___ | ___ | ___ |

Core and agility exercise circuit:

Speed skaters – 3 sets for 30 seconds

Bicycles (abs) – 3 sets of 12+ repetitions

Bird dogs – 3 sets of 30 seconds per side (i.e., 60 seconds total per set)

General stretching

**Day 2:** _____

Five minute warm-up

General stretching

| Resistance exercise circuit: | Set 1 | Set 2 | Set 3 | Set 4 |
|---|---|---|---|---|
| Dead lifts | ___/___ | ___/___ | ___/___ | ___/___ |
| Shoulder press | ___/___ | ___/___ | ___/___ | ___/___ |
| Lawnmowers (one-arm rows) | ___/___ | ___/___ | ___/___ | ___/___ |

Circuit core and agility exercises:

Medicine ball toes taps – 3 sets of 40 to 50 repetitions per foot

Anchored abdominal raises – 3 sets of 12+ repetitions

Lying back extensions – 3 sets of 60 seconds total

General stretching

# WEEK 1:

**Day 3:** _____

Five minute warm-up

General stretching

High intensity workout (for time):

 ¼ mile run on treadmill, 20 body weight squats, 12 pushups

 ½ mile run on treadmill, 20 body weight squats, 12 pushups

 ¾ mile run on treadmill, 20 body weight squats, 12 pushups

 ½ mile run on treadmill, 20 body weight squats, 12 pushups

 ¼ mile run on treadmill

Time: _____

General stretching


**Day 4:** _____

Five minute warm-up

General stretching

| Resistance exercise circuit: | Set 1 | Set 2 | Set 3 | Set 4 |
|---|---|---|---|---|
| Thrusters | ___/___ | ___/___ | ___/___ | ___/___ |
| Curls to shoulder presses | ___/___ | ___/___ | ___/___ | ___/___ |
| Dips (reps) | ___ | ___ | ___ | ___ |

Circuit core and agility exercises:

 180 surfers – 45 seconds, 3 sets

 Jumps – 10 repetitions, 3 sets

 Front and side planks – 45 seconds, 3 sets

General stretching

# WEEK 2:

**Day 1:** _____

Five minute warm-up

| Resistance exercise circuit: | Set 1 | Set 2 | Set 3 | Set 4 |
|---|---|---|---|---|
| Walking lunges | ___/___ | ___/___ | ___/___ | ___/___ |
| Upright rows | ___/___ | ___/___ | ___/___ | ___/___ |
| Chest press/bench press | ___/___ | ___/___ | ___/___ | ___/___ |

Circuit core and agility exercises:

Adductions and Abductions – 3 sets of 15 repetitions per exercise per leg

Moth to cocoons – 3 sets of 12+ repetitions

Lying back extensions – 3 sets of 60 seconds total

General stretching


**Day 2:** _____

Five minute warm-up

General stretching

| Resistance exercise circuit: | Set 1 | Set 2 | Set 3 | Set 4 |
|---|---|---|---|---|
| Power cleans | ___/___ | ___/___ | ___/___ | ___/___ |
| Push ups | ___ | ___ | ___ | ___ |
| Lat pulley rows | ___/___ | ___/___ | ___/___ | ___/___ |

Core and agility exercise circuit:

Swing kicks – 3 sets of 12 repetitions

Anchored abdominal raises – 3 sets of 12+ repetitions

Bird dogs – 3 sets of 30 seconds per side

General stretching

# WEEK 2:

**Day 3:** _____

Five minute warm-up

General stretching

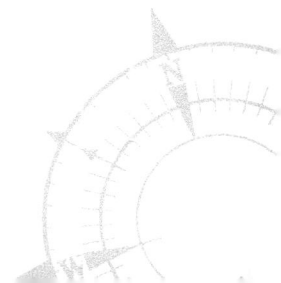

High intensity workout (for time):

 Treadmill for ¼ mile, 20 dead lifts, 6 pull ups

 Treadmill for ½ mile, 20 dead lifts, 6 pull ups

 Treadmill for 1mile, 20 dead lifts, 6 pull ups

 Treadmill for ½ mile, 20 dead lifts, 6 pull ups

 Treadmill for ¼ mile

Time: _____

General stretching


**Day 4:** _____

Five minute warm-up

General stretching

| Resistance exercise circuit: | Set 1 | Set 2 | Set 3 | Set 4 |
|---|---|---|---|---|
| Cleans to thrusts | ___/___ | ___/___ | ___/___ | ___/___ |
| Pull ups/lat pull downs | ___/___ | ___/___ | ___/___ | ___/___ |
| Push ups | ___ | ___ | ___ | ___ |

Circuit core and agility exercises:

 Single leg hops – 3 sets of 10 reps with each leg, each

  direction

 Step ups – 3 sets for 45 seconds

 Bicycles – 3 sets of 12+ repetitions

 Straight leg dead lifts – 3 sets of 12+ repetitions

General stretching

# WEEK 3:

**Day 1:** _____

Five minute warm-up

General stretching

| Resistance exercise circuit: | Set 1 | Set 2 | Set 3 | Set 4 |
|---|---|---|---|---|
| Thrusters | ___/___ | ___/___ | ___/___ | ___/___ |
| Dips | ___ | ___ | ___ | ___ |
| Lat pulley rows | ___/___ | ___/___ | ___/___ | ___/___ |

Core and agility exercise circuit:

Medicine ball wall tosses – 3 sets for 60 seconds

Anchored abdominal raises – 3 sets of 12+ repetitions

Bird dogs – 3 sets for 30 seconds per side

General stretching

**Day 2:** _____

Five minute warm-up

General stretching

| Resistance exercise circuit: | Set 1 | Set 2 | Set 3 | Set 4 |
|---|---|---|---|---|
| Squats | ___/___ | ___/___ | ___/___ | ___/___ |
| Curls to shoulder presses | ___/___ | ___/___ | ___/___ | ___/___ |
| Upright rows | ___/___ | ___/___ | ___/___ | ___/___ |

Circuit core and agility exercises:

Sideways runs – 3 sets of 4 laps

Moth to cocoons – 3 sets of 12+ repetitions

Lying back extensions – 3 sets of 60 seconds total

General stretching

# WEEK 3:

**Day 3:** _____

Five minute warm-up

General stretching

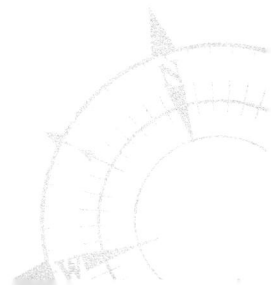

High intensity workout (for time):

    ½ mile run on treadmill, 3 minutes on bike – fast pace, 12 pushups

    ½ mile run on treadmill, 3 minutes on bike – fast pace, 12 pushups

    ½ mile run on treadmill, 3 minutes on bike – fast pace, 12 pushups

    ½ mile run on treadmill

Time: _____

General stretching


**Day 4:** _____

Five minute warm-up

General stretching

| Resistance exercise circuit: | Set 1 | Set 2 | Set 3 | Set 4 |
|---|---|---|---|---|
| Dead lifts | ___/___ | ___/___ | ___/___ | ___/___ |
| Pull ups/lat pull downs | ___/___ | ___/___ | ___/___ | ___/___ |
| Chest press/bench press | ___/___ | ___/___ | ___/___ | ___/___ |

Circuit core and agility exercises:

    Medicine ball toe taps – 50 repetitions per foot, 3 sets

    Calf leans – 30 seconds, 3 sets

    Front and side planks – 45 seconds, 3 sets

General stretching

# WEEK 4:

**Day 1:** _____

Five minute warm-up

General stretching

| Resistance exercise circuit: | Set 1 | Set 2 | Set 3 | Set 4 |
|---|---|---|---|---|
| Power cleans | __/__ | __/__ | __/__ | __/__ |
| Lawnmowers (one-arm rows) | __/__ | __/__ | __/__ | __/__ |
| Push ups | __ | __ | __ | __ |

Circuit core and agility exercises:

Speed skaters – 3 sets of 45 seconds

Bicycles – 3 sets of 12+ repetitions

Straight leg dead lifts – 3 sets of 12+ repetitions

General stretching


**Day 2:** _____

Five minute warm-up

General stretching

| Resistance exercise circuit: | Set 1 | Set 2 | Set 3 | Set 4 |
|---|---|---|---|---|
| Push presses | __/__ | __/__ | __/__ | __/__ |
| Lat pulley rows | __/__ | __/__ | __/__ | __/__ |
| Dips | __ | __ | __ | __ |

Circuit core and agility exercises:

Single leg hops– 3 sets of 10 repetitions with each foot, each direction

180 surfers – 3 sets of 30 seconds

Anchored abdominal raises – 3 sets of 12+ repetitions

Bird dogs – 3 sets of 30 seconds per side

General stretching

# WEEK 4:

**Day 3:** _____

Five minute warm-up

General stretching

High intensity workout (for time):

     15 dead lifts, 15 upright rows, 15 shoulder presses

     14 dead lifts, 14 upright rows, 14 shoulder presses

     13 dead lifts, 13 upright rows, 13 shoulder presses

     ……..

     1 dead lift, 1 upright row, 1 shoulder press

Never let the bar touch the ground

Time: _____

General stretching


**Day 4:** _____

Five minute warm-up

General stretching

| Resistance exercise circuit: | Set 1 | Set 2 | Set 3 | Set 4 |
|---|---|---|---|---|
| Squats | ___/___ | ___/___ | ___/___ | ___/___ |
| Lat pull downs/pull ups | ___/___ | ___/___ | ___/___ | ___/___ |
| Chest press/benchpress | ___/___ | ___/___ | ___/___ | ___/___ |

Circuit core and agility exercises:

    Agility runs – 3 sets of 3 laps

    Jump ups – 3 sets of 30 seconds

    Front and side planks – 3 sets of 45 seconds

General stretching

As you look over this program, several patterns should emerge.

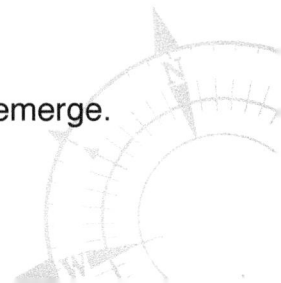

# WEEK 5:

**Day 1:** _____

Five minute warm-up

General stretching

| Resistance exercise circuit: | Set 1 | Set 2 | Set 3 | Set 4 |
|---|---|---|---|---|
| Walking lunges | __/__ | __/__ | __/__ | __/__ |
| Lat pulley rows | __/__ | __/__ | __/__ | __/__ |
| Curl to shoulder presses | __/__ | __/__ | __/__ | __/__ |

Circuit core and agility exercises:

180 surfers – 3 sets of 30 seconds

Moth to cocoons – 3 sets of 12+ repetitions

Lying back extensions – 3 sets for 10 seconds per side (60 seconds total each set)

General stretching


**Day 2:** _____

Five minute warm-up

General stretching

| Resistance exercise circuit: | Set 1 | Set 2 | Set 3 | Set 4 |
|---|---|---|---|---|
| Dead lifts | __/__ | __/__ | __/__ | __/__ |
| Upright rows | __/__ | __/__ | __/__ | __/__ |
| Pushups | __ | __ | __ | __ |

Circuit core and agility exercises:

Medicine ball toe taps – 3 sets of 50 repetitions per foot

Bicycles – 3 sets of 12+ repetitions

Bird dogs – 3 sets of 30 seconds per side (60 seconds total)

General stretching

# WEEK 5:

**Day 3:** _____

Five minute warm-up

General stretching

High intensity workout (for time):

¼ mile run on treadmill, 20 body weight squats, 12 pushups

½ mile run on treadmill, 20 body weight squats, 12 pushups

¾ mile run on treadmill, 20 body weight squats, 12 pushups

½ mile run on treadmill, 20 body weight squats, 12 pushups

¼ mile run on treadmill

Time: _____

General stretching


**Day 4:** _____

Five minute warm-up

General stretching

| Resistance exercise circuit: | Set 1 | Set 2 | Set 3 | Set 4 |
|---|---|---|---|---|
| Power cleans | ___/___ | ___/___ | ___/___ | ___/___ |
| Dips | ___ | ___ | ___ | ___ |
| Lawn mowers (one arm rows) | ___/___ | ___/___ | ___/___ | ___/___ |

Circuit core and agility exercises:

Speed skaters – 3 sets of 30 seconds

Calf leans – 3 sets of 30 seconds

Anchored abdominal raises – 3 sets of 12+ repetitions

Straight leg dead lifts – 3 sets of 12+ repetitions

General stretching

# WEEK 6:

**Day 1:** _____

Five minute warm-up

General stretching

| Resistance exercise circuit: | Set 1 | Set 2 | Set 3 | Set 4 |
|---|---|---|---|---|
| Thrusters | ___/___ | ___/___ | ___/___ | ___/___ |
| Pull ups/pull downs | ___/___ | ___/___ | ___/___ | ___/___ |
| Chest press/bench press | ___/___ | ___/___ | ___/___ | ___/___ |

Circuit core and agility exercises:

    Jump ups – 3 sets of 10 repetitions

    Swing kicks – 3 sets of 12 repetitions

    Front and side planks – 3 sets of 45 seconds

General stretching

**Day 2:** _____

Five minute warm-up

General stretching

| Resistance exercise circuit: | Set 1 | Set 2 | Set 3 | Set 4 |
|---|---|---|---|---|
| Squats | ___/___ | ___/___ | ___/___ | ___/___ |
| Lat pulley rows | ___/___ | ___/___ | ___/___ | ___/___ |
| Push press | ___ | ___ | ___ | ___ |

Circuit core and agility exercises:

    Single leg hops– 3 sets of 8 repetitions with each foot

    Sideways runs – 3 sets of 4 laps

    Bicycles – 3 sets of 12+ repetitions

    Lying back extensions – 3 sets of 30 seconds per side

General stretching

# WEEK 6:

**Day 3:** _____

Five minute warm-up

General stretching

High intensity workout (for time):

    Tabata sets – 20 seconds on, 10 second rest for a total of 4

    minutes (8 mini-sets)

        Tabata squats (body weight or light weight, e.g. medicine ball)

        Tabata upright rows

        Tabata push ups

        Tabata bicycles

        Tabata straight leg dead lifts

Time: _____

General stretching


**Day 4:** _____

Five minute warm-up

General stretching

| Resistance exercise circuit: | Set 1 | Set 2 | Set 3 | Set 4 |
|---|---|---|---|---|
| Walking lunges | ___/___ | ___/___ | ___/___ | ___/___ |
| Shoulder press | ___/___ | ___/___ | ___/___ | ___/___ |
| Pull ups/pull downs | ___/___ | ___/___ | ___/___ | ___/___ |

Circuit core and agility exercises:

    Medicine ball toe taps – 3 sets of 50 reps per foot

    Moth to cocoons – 3 sets of 12+ repetitions

    Bird dogs – 3 sets of 30 seconds per side

General stretching

Several themes in this programming appear. The first is that, while there is little repetition of exercises and no repeated routines, many of the workouts contain full body resistance movements that span numerous joints and require the control of an external object (e.g., a barbell, dumbbell, or medicine ball). These full body movements certainly require and develop muscle and bone strength. In addition, due to the recruitment of several large muscle groups, significant oxygen is required to meet metabolic demands, thus both the aerobic and anaerobic pathways are utilized and trained. Further, due to the need to generate and control the transfer of momentum from one part of the body to another (generally large muscles to smaller muscles), the core is actively engaged as a stabilizer and significant balance is required. Finally, by performing these movements through their full range of motion, flexibility is enhanced.

A second pattern is the inclusion of heavy weight work such as barbell squats, dead lifts, and bench press as well as lighter weight resistance work using one's body weight or a medicine ball. The heavy load work requires significant effort over a shorter duration, thus focusing on the anaerobic metabolic pathways. The lighter load

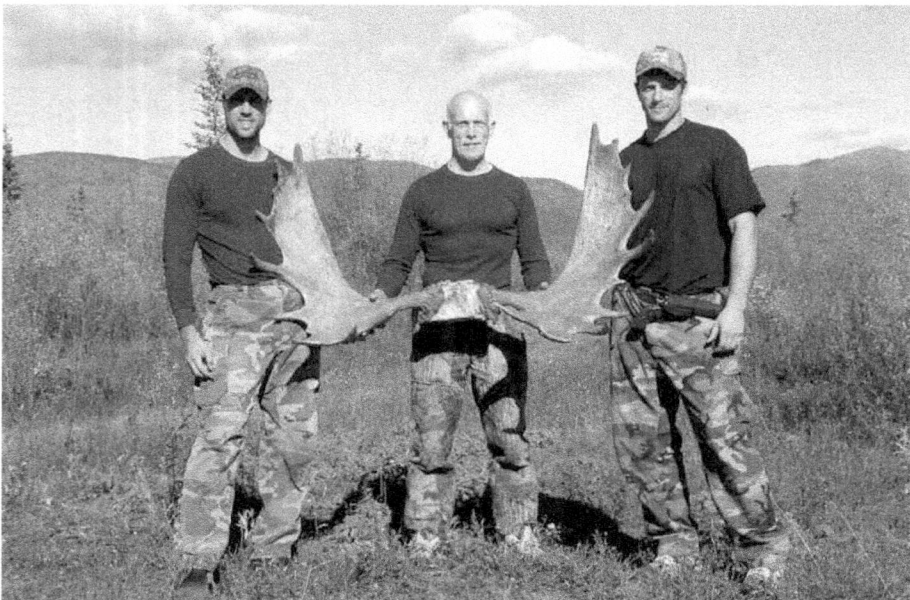

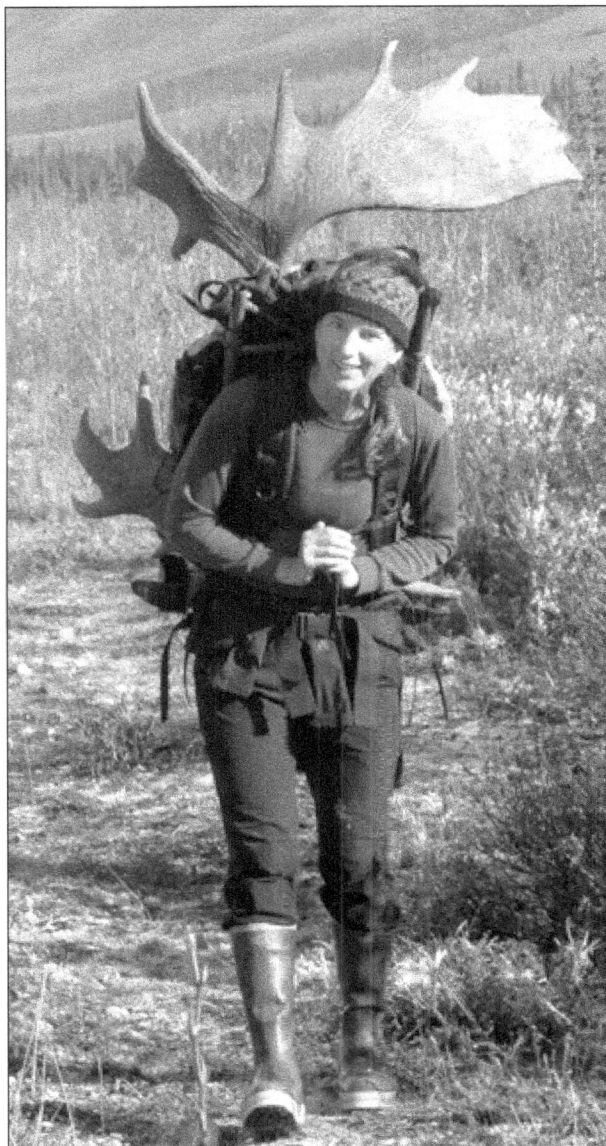

work can be performed at an increased pace per repetition or for a longer duration. This approach will focus on muscular endurance and provide both aerobic and anaerobic benefits.

Third, many of the resistance exercises are performed in a circuit. This allows reduced down time as one muscle group is recovering as another is being trained. The overall intensity can be managed through the amount of rest between sets of exercises. This approach elevates heart rate throughout the resistance portion of the workout, thus blurring the lines between "weights" and "cardio". This decompartmentalization is both efficient and practical.

A fourth pattern is a crafted balance in the selection of the resistance exercises such that a "push" exercise is balanced with a "pull" exercise. For example, pull ups may be paired with dips. This is directly counter to the compartmental approach of "back" days and "chest" days. In essence, within any given workout, most of the body is actively engaged at one point or another.

A fifth pattern is the frequent and specific inclusion of exercises that explicitly challenge one's balance, coordination, and agility, typical components of most strenuous outdoor activities. Almost every client I have worked with has been largely undertrained in these components of fitness. However, this is the training area where they have seen the most dramatic improvement, the most practical trans-ferability outside the gym, and identify as the most fun. An additional benefit of this work is that, if performed at high intensity with limited rest, cardiovascular endurance can be enhanced. Perhaps the most compelling reason to train for balance, coordination, and agility is their direct link to one's physical confidence. My clients have quickly changed their mindset relative to certain activities from "I can't do that" to "I'll give it a try" to "let's do it again, only higher or faster".

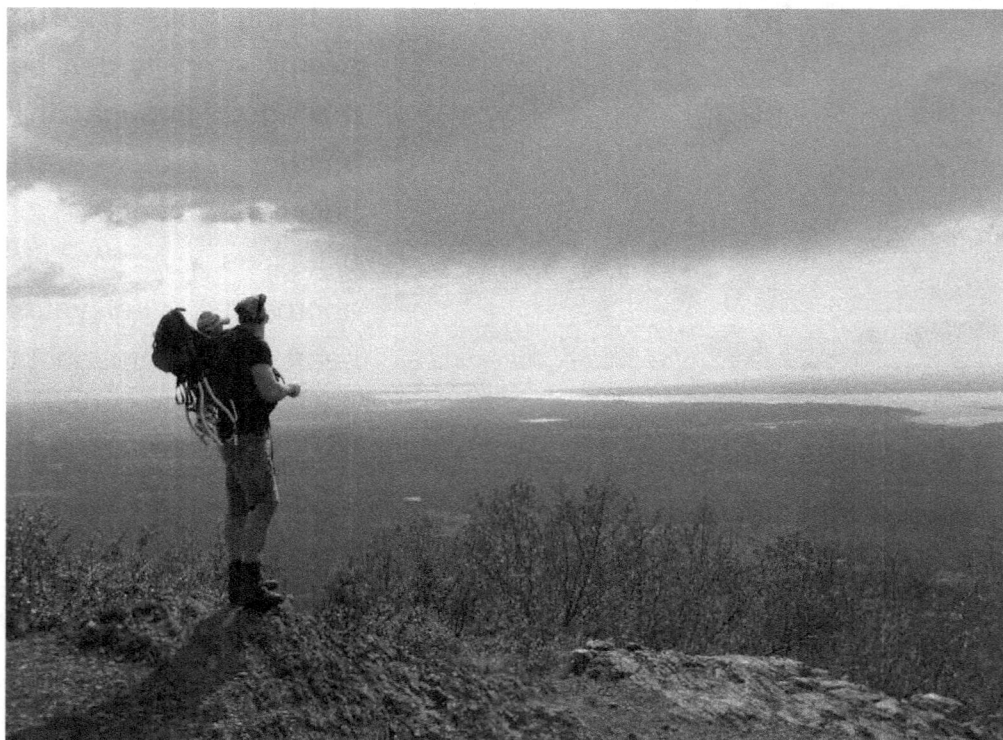

A sixth pattern is the prescription for warming up and stretching before and after each session. This helps prepare the body for the work ahead by elevating body temperature and increasing heart rate. Most importantly, the pre-workout stretch, in concert with proper form, can prevent muscle, ligament, or tendon injuries. The post-workout stretch, coupled with exercises performed through a full range of motion will improve flexibility. Stretching and warming up is an extra chore before those dark early morning trips to the duck blind, but it will make the entire day seem to go easier, particularly as flexibility tends to decline with age.

A seventh pattern is the inclusion of rest days. I recommend training only four to five days per week. The rest days should be spent on recreational activities or recuperating, but not on additional training sessions. Rest means rest. Take it easy. Your body needs to recuperate and recharge periodically. Tune up and organize your equipment, read your journals or other materials to stay in the mindset of hurting or fishing, or just spend some time outdoors.

A final pattern is the occasional timed workout that serves to set benchmarks and monitor achievement through time by assessing performance across the majority of fitness categories.

When approached this way, it is obvious that there are a limitless number of workouts than can be crafted. The art lies in constructing workouts that are constantly varied (in part to maintain interest) and span the categories of fitness widely. The science requires that the exercises are balanced, performed at high intensity, and include warm-ups and stretching each session.

*"Your body is designed
to handle and utilize
high quality, nutritious,
whole foods"*

# CHAPTER 10:

## NUTRITION

FIT 4 THE FIELD

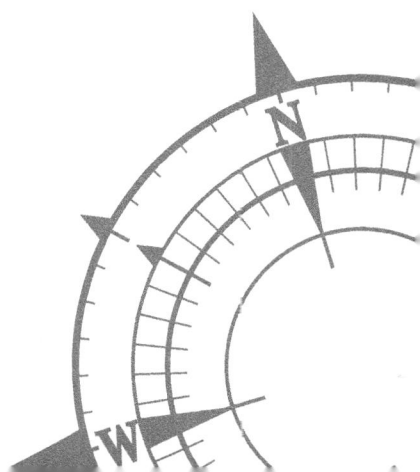

Early in my career as a wildlife biologist, I largely specialized in nutrition. As I monitored indi-vidual animals and populations, the importance of food was readily apparent. Obtaining and consuming the necessary quantity and quality of calories was the difference between starvation and survival. Nutrition further impacted the ability of individual animals to produce and support offspring. This productivity, when viewed at the population level determined if the population would increase, decrease, or remain stable. This information, in part, determined the number of animals available for human harvest.

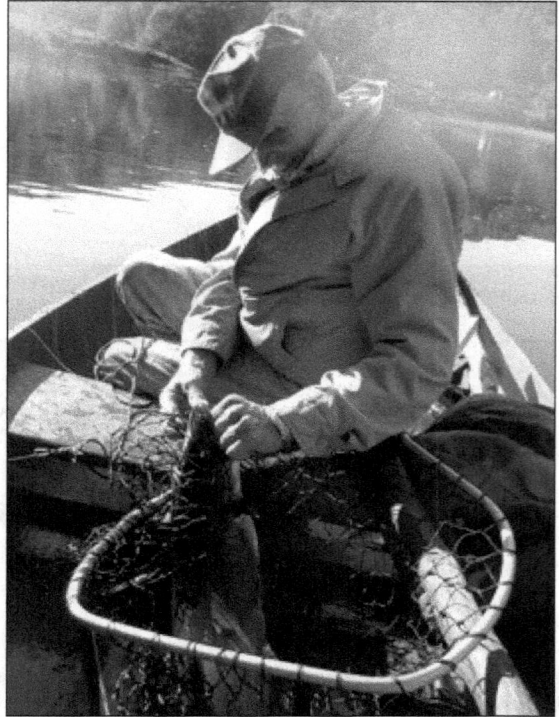

Humans in much of the developed world have a different relationship with food. More often than not, people are looking to lose weight for health, aesthetic, or performance purposes. Unfortunately, the "diet" industry dominates much of the information available through the media leading to confusion and false expectations. There are no short cuts for good decisions and hard work.

When you are training to optimize your physical performance proper nutrition is critical. The nutrients we consume serve as the raw materials and fuel that maintain our body and support our training efforts and recreational activities. Providing our body with adequate and appropriate nutrients is of paramount importance.

When working with clients I strive to simplify the many conflicting messages that barrage all of us relative to diet and nutrition. I also tend to stress moderation in all things. My general recommendations are summarized below:

**Point 1:** Avoid "Diets"– strive to develop healthy habits you can maintain every day for the rest of your life.

**Point 2:** Be patient. Expect major changes in body compositions (e.g., gaining 5 lbs of muscle or losing 20+ lbs of body fat) to take a year. You are better off doing it "the right way" rather than "the fast way".

**Point 3:** Eat consciously – be aware of what you eat. Avoid eating in front of the TV, in the car, or while working on the computer.

**Point 4:** Control portion size. Leave some empty space on your plate.

**Point 5:** Don't automatically take seconds, allow 20 minutes to pass. If you are still hungry, take about 1/3 the amount of your original portion.

**Point 6:** Fresh, local fruit and vegetables are best. Select frozen over canned.

**Point 7:** Select organics when you can. Better yet, grow, pick, and harvest your own.

**Point 8:** Choose color...select red, green, yellow, and orange vegetables in addition to or instead of white carbohydrates.

**Point 9:** Choose whole grains over processed flours. The closer to the earth, the better.

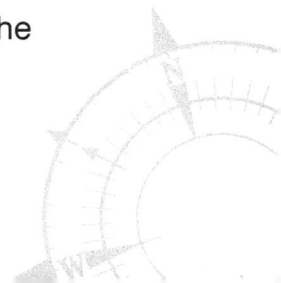

**Point 10:** Don't shop hungry. Shop the outside aisles of the store first. This is where the perishable (and therefore, more healthy) items are located. This will ensure that your impulse buys will be better for you.

**Point 11:** Minimize processed sugars. Limit sodas, go for one package instead of two in your coffee and tea, and minimize candy consumption.

**Point 12:** Hydrate and keep alcohol and caffeine consumption moderate.

**Point 13:** Don't fear fats – they are necessary and important parts of a healthy diet. Just focus on quality fats found in fish, nuts, olive oil, etc.

**Point 14:** Avoid fast food and eat smart when eating out. When possible, look at grilled chicken and fish, salads, or vegetarian options.

**Point 15:** Small changes add up…select 2% milk rather than half and half, get the 6 oz steak instead of the 10 oz steak, substitute double churned or light ice cream/frozen yogurt (remember portion control!) for the high-sugar/high fat options, get the whole grain rice as a side instead of the fries, go with dark chocolate with a cocoa content >70%.

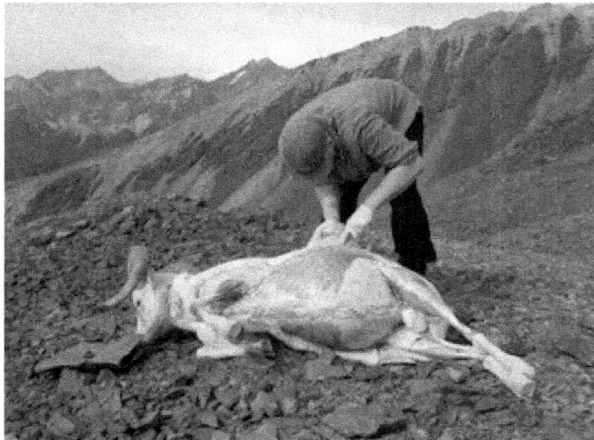

**Point 16:** Keep a food journal for one month. Awareness will lead to more informed decisions

**Point 17:** Pay attention to your cravings and your body. Consuming quality calories before your blood sugar drops will reduce over-consumption or binging on low-quality calories.

**Point 18:** Plan ahead...poor planning leads to limited options.

**Point 19:** Don't stress... you simply want to make more good choices than poor choices. Though time, you will find that healthy choices will lead to healthy cravings.

**Point 20:** Enjoy food! Food is your friend, not the enemy so it is important you keep a positive relationship with what you eat.

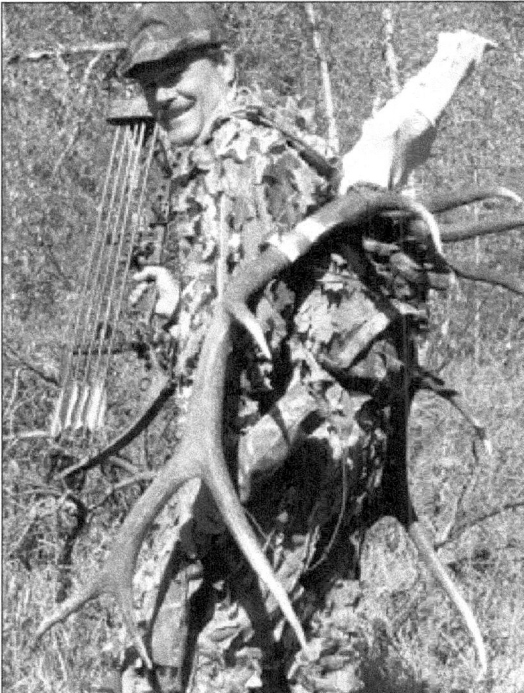

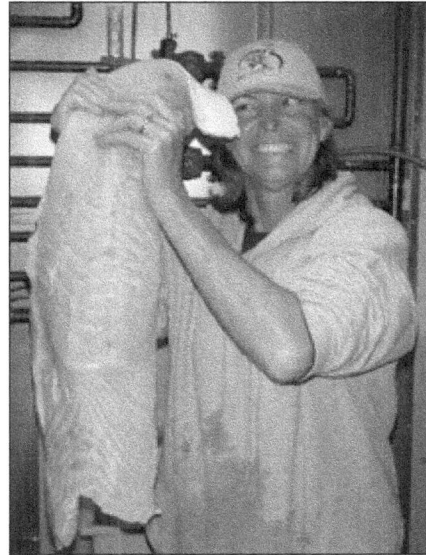

# SYNTHESIS

Our connection to the outdoors is undeniable. Our innate desire to hunt, fish, hike, take photos, or just enjoy a sunset or summer evening breeze are evidence that we were simply meant to do these things. Further, these activities are central to our fundamental social unit, the family, as they have been from our collective beginning. They are part of what bonds us together, what we all have in common.

Taking care of ourselves physically is critical to ensuring our emotional and spiritual well-being throughout our lives as this allows us to participate in the activities we cherish. Unlike many athletic pursuits, outdoor recreation is a lifelong endeavor, one you can actively share with your children and grandchildren. The skills, knowledge, and memories you share with your family are part of your heritage. The example you set is part of your legacy.

The intent of this guide is to provide you a path to enhance and maintain your fitness throughout the seasons and throughout your life, to maximize your memories, and expand your horizons. I wish you well in all of your adventures yet to come.

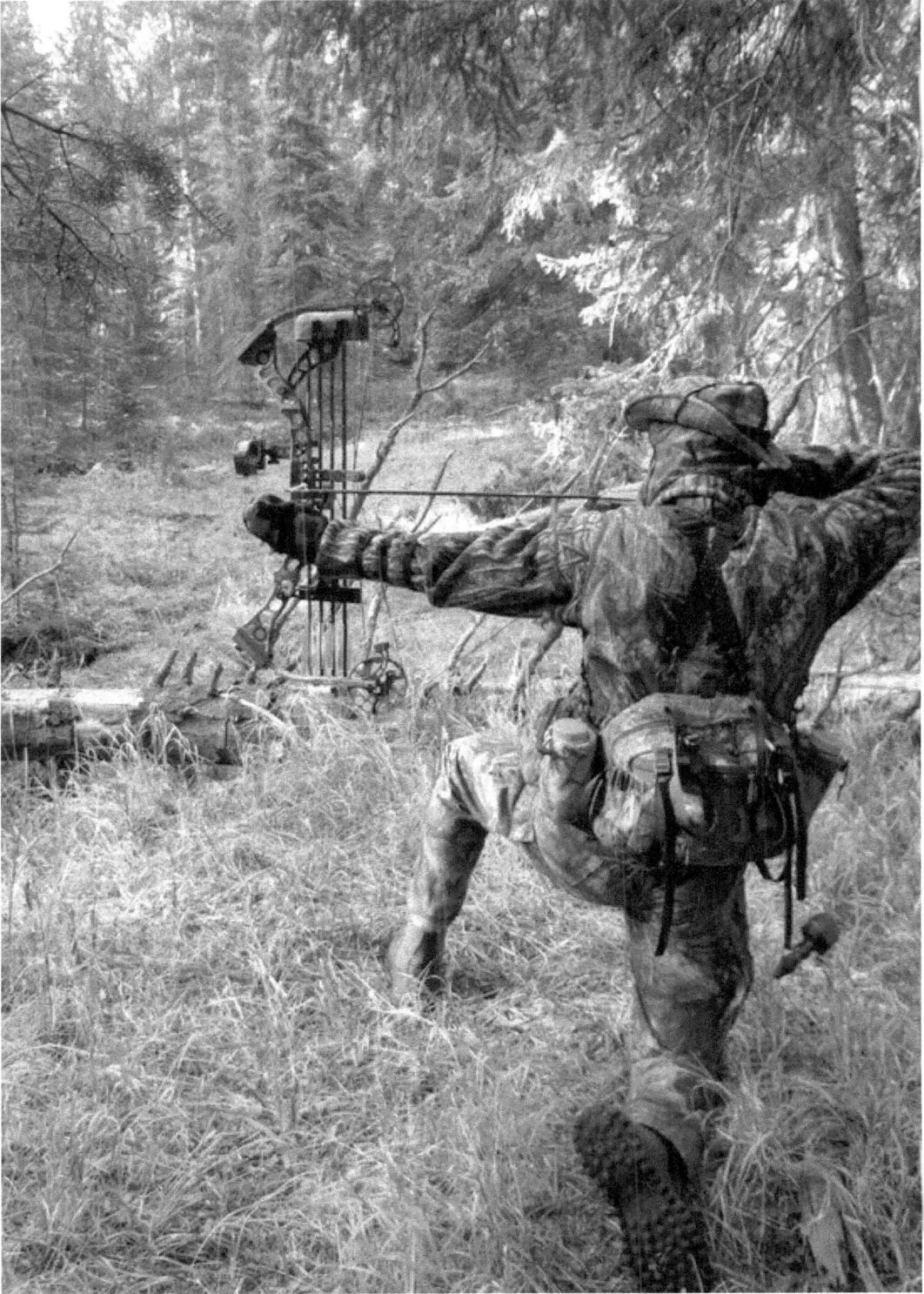

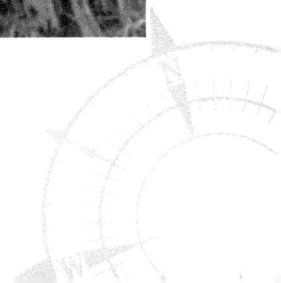

www.ingramcontent.com/pod-product-compliance
Lightning Source LLC
Chambersburg PA
CBHW081156270326
41930CB00014B/3173